Praise for *Through the Flames*

"This is a riveting tale that begins with the sort of unimaginable tragedy that lurks in our darkest nightmares. But instead of a journey of suffering and pain, Allan Lokos offers up a memoir of recovery that becomes a glorious display of fortitude, resilience, and wisdom. Lokos was chosen, it seems, to personally answer the question wrestled with for centuries by everyone from Buddhist scholars to meditation neophytes: can the practice of mindfulness and meditation actually allow the human spirit to triumph over extreme and unimpeachable suffering? Yes, his story tells us. And it offers lessons in courage, humor, and compassion for the rest of us as well. I was transfixed and couldn't put it down. It is stunning and inspiring."
> —Claire Shipman, ABC News reporter and *New York Times*–bestselling author of *The Confidence Code* and *Womenomics*

"'Once burnt, twice shy,' the saying goes. And yet, *Through the Flames* proves that his heart-rending fiery ordeal made Allan Lokos twice as courageous, twice as determined, patient, and compassionate. His story—utterly fascinating and inspiring—makes us want to imitate his admirable way of coping. Indeed he offers us solid practical advice on how to go through the flames we ourselves must endure to come out more like the persons we deep down want to be. A treasure of wisdom and compassion awaits you between the covers of this book."
> —Brother David Steindl-Rast, Benedictine monk, author and spiritual teacher, and cofounder of Gratefulness.org

"In *Through the Flames*, Allan Lokos shares his personal suffering while healing from a traumatic injury. His story brings us closer to the wisdom and the determination we all have within us to live life deeply. This book is on the one hand a story of our common bond in suffering and the other a new and refreshing opportunity to learn from a master the practical ways meditation, patience, and self-compassion can help us live."
> —Amy Acton, executive director, Phoenix Society for Burn Survivors

"In this heartfelt and unflinching memoir, Allan Lokos gives a lucid account of how Buddhist practice enabled him to come to terms with a life suddenly interrupted by a violent accident and its aftermath. *Through the Flames* is an inspiration."
> —Stephen Batchelor, author of *Confession of a Buddhist Atheist* and *Buddhism without Beliefs*

THROUGH
THE FLAMES

THROUGH THE FLAMES

Overcoming Disaster through Compassion, Patience, and Determination

ALLAN LOKOS

JEREMY P. TARCHER/PENGUIN

a member of Penguin Group (USA)

New York

JEREMY P. TARCHER/PENGUIN
Published by the Penguin Group
Penguin Group (USA) LLC
375 Hudson Street
New York, New York 10014

USA · Canada · UK · Ireland · Australia
New Zealand · India · South Africa · China

penguin.com
A Penguin Random House Company

Most Tarcher/Penguin books are available at special quantity discounts for
bulk purchase for sales promotions, premiums, fund-raising, and educational needs.
Special books or book excerpts also can be created to fit specific needs.
For details, write: Special.Markets@us.penguingroup.com.

ISBN: 978-0-399-17180-2

Printed in the United States of America
1   3   5   7   9   10   8   6   4   2

BOOK DESIGN BY TANYA MAIBORODA

For

THE COMMUNITY MEDITATION CENTER

A sacred illness is one that educates us
and alters us from the inside out,
provides experiences and therefore knowledge
that we could not possibly achieve in any other way,
and aligns us with a life path that is, ultimately,
of benefit to ourselves and those around us.

——DEENA METZGER
Poet, novelist, essayist, storyteller,
teacher, healer, and medicine woman
b. 1936, BROOKLYN, NEW YORK

CONTENTS

FOREWORD

Once, when I was being interviewed for a magazine article, the journalist tossed an unexpected question at me. "What is the role of mindfulness or meditation at a time of complete crisis?" The words I heard come out of my mouth spontaneously in response: "I wouldn't wait."

Of course, some people do wait for the bottom to fall out from under them, for an emergency, for some kind of disaster before they reach for a resource like mindfulness, and even then it may well provide some support.

But if we can strengthen mindfulness in times of more ordinary stress and challenge, in a regular day, the qualities that come from mindfulness—compassion, balance, awareness, and openness—develop as a kind of muscle memory that accompanies us right into times of great fear, despair, or upheaval. These qualities reveal some sense of what is intact and whole within us, no matter what. They bring us back to the essential aspects of ourselves, like the capacity to love, which cannot be destroyed, even if everything else somehow does feel like it already has been or may well soon be destroyed.

Now, and I suspect for the rest of my life, whenever I think of that response, "I wouldn't wait," I picture Allan Lokos and his wife, Susanna Weiss.

Having done so much of my meditation training with Burmese teachers, and feeling such a strong affinity for the country, I follow a few different sources of Burmese news on Twitter. I saw right away the reports of a plane crash on Christmas Day 2012. I knew several people in Burma at the time, but I didn't see any reports of Americans injured or killed. I watched some You-Tube videos of Australians who had been on the plane who seemed perfectly okay. What I didn't consider was just how much depended on where on the airplane your seat was.

A few days after the crash, I got an e-mail from Susanna, saying she and Allan had been on that plane. At that point, they were in Bangkok. From the time of that e-mail onward, I had the chance to bear witness to the ever-shifting, kaleidoscopic picture of the new world of injury, trauma, resilience, and healing they had entered.

Through the Flames recounts Allan's depiction of the crash and what follows, via the lens of his own experience, and for the immediate experience and aftermath, what he has gleaned from Susanna and medical records, and via the perspectives of others. It is also the story of the mindfulness, balance, and compassion Allan brought forth from within himself to meet the intensity and shock and pain of the moment, first in order to survive, then in order to recover, and ultimately to flourish. It is the story of the patience and the kindness we are all capable of, no matter who we are or what we go through. It is the story of the incredible resilience of the human spirit and the fact that we can each learn how to access and trust it.

More than anything, *Through the Flames* seems to me to be a love story. It is the story of Allan and Susanna's love for each other. It is the story of the love for humankind displayed by medical personnel. It is the story of the love of friends who will go the extra mile to help out someone who needs them. It is the story of the extraordinary, grace-filled love of life Allan demonstrates, a love that is so much bigger than any circumstance.

We probably all know people who go through pain or suffering and get ensnared in a sense of isolation, bitterness, or self-loathing. Seeing someone right in the midst of their vulnerability and distress turn again and again to awareness, love, and compassion is inspiring beyond words.

Recently, a friend ran into Allan and saw how calm, kind, and at ease Allan seems these days. He put it succinctly: "You can't see Allan without thinking his recovery is nothing short of a miracle."

I phrase it like that myself sometimes. But in truth, most often, when I think of what Allan and Susanna have gone through, when I think of what we so often go through in our lives—the tremendous joys and the sorrows and everything in between—and the potential we have for understanding, for awareness, and for love, I find that I fundamentally and repeatedly come back to, "Practice now, strengthen those qualities right now. I wouldn't wait."

—*Sharon Salzberg*

INTRODUCTION

This tale is one that, until the end of 2012, I would never have imagined writing. After all, one should have the appropriate knowledge and experience to write about a specific subject. I can honestly say that I wish I did not have the experience or background. Yet the thought that sharing the unimaginable and terrifying event that I lived through could be of benefit to others inspires and motivates me.

I wanted to present the details as accurately as possible with no exaggeration, no aggrandizement, and no "poetic license." In order to do so, I had to rely heavily upon my wife, Susanna, since much of the time described in part one, "Christmas," I was unconscious, dazed, in shock, or in a drug-induced state. Even when I was awake, my memories, particularly of the first few weeks, would have to be viewed as unreliable. Susanna was with me through just about every minute offered herein. She was definitely awake and aware. She had to be if I was to survive. Fortunately, she is bright, articulate, and usually imperturbable. I believe that between us we have produced an authentic account. Truth does not need embellishment.

I began taking notes for this narrative in April 2013, and wrote the actual manuscript from June 2013 through March 2014. I did most of the "writing" with dictation software, which was essentially a new experience for me. (The reason for the dictation method will soon be evident.)

Since I had written my previous books, articles, and stories using the more standard computer and keyboard method, I was concerned that my brain-to-speech process might not work as well as my more familiar brain-to-hands process. I found the dictation method amazing, frustrating, and amusing: amazing because it actually works, frustrating because of how often it does not, and amusing because of what it creates when it falters. As an example, "Myanmar" (Burma) became "Me and Ma." We battled endlessly over the spelling of my first name, with me clinging desperately to that which was chosen by my parents so many years ago, while it created numerous clever and innovative alternatives. Even so, I remain amazed at how all my spoken words became zeros and ones, and they in turn became printed words, all in less time than it takes to say "Me and Ma." Nevertheless, I got the hang of it and began to find the process quite seductive.

THE CORE significance of dukkha (Sanskrit: suffering, stress) in Buddhist thought has led some casual observers to suggest that Buddhism is a pessimistic ideology. The emphasis on dukkha, however, when viewed as intended, does not present a negative view but rather a practical and realistic assessment of the human condition. The Buddhist view is that all beings experience suffering. This includes, but by no means is limited to, sickness, old age, and death. It incorporates every moment of dissatisfaction, unhappiness, discomfort, displeasure, and more. Dukkha is intricately interwoven with the joys, delights, and beauty of everyday life. The most accurate appraisal of the Buddhist philosophy is that it is neither pessimistic nor optimistic, but realistic.

The reality is that what happened to me is unlikely to happen to you. If it did, just like me, it is highly improbable that you would survive. I was just fortunate/blessed/lucky/being watched over, or as the Buddhists might say, the conditions did not quite come together to bring about my demise.

All of us experience dukkha. I have lived through some of the most challenging dukkha imaginable and have managed to maintain, and in some ways improve upon, a previously wonderful life. I have been asked again and again how I have done that. I do not want to mislead—it has often been a struggle beyond what I ever could have imagined. There were days when it felt as if the mountain was just too formidable for this mere mortal to climb.

SOMETIMES WE dismiss the counsel of others because we feel that they could not possibly understand; no one could understand. We feel we are absolutely alone: *No one has ever had to endure what I am going through.* While there is some truth to that lonely perspective, I believe that the greater, more accurate view, and certainly the more beneficial view, is that we are in this together. I assure you that I have been in the fire with you and I have come through the flames.

The ensuing narrative may appear to be about one person's journey, but in truth it is about reality; the reality of suffering; its cause; and a path that can lead to its cessation. It is my chosen path, and just as I have had to carve out a trail for myself, you will have to do the same for yourself. My hope is that my experience might serve as a guide.

In part one, "Christmas," we start out enjoying a holiday but end up in a nightmare, a devastating event occurring thousands of miles from home. Professional opinions in Myanmar (Burma), Bangkok, and Singapore were that I could not possibly survive. Back home in New York City the prognosis was the same. Fortunately for me, they were wrong.

The writing of "Christmas," the first section of this book, was a stressful endeavor and at times quite upsetting. While acknowledging that parts of this story were difficult to write, I also want to mention that there may be those for whom "Christmas," in particular, could be difficult to read. Please be wise, and when necessary, slow down and/or take a break.

Part two, "Healing," moves through the travails of surviving all the way to thriving, acknowledging, among other diverse phenomena, the extraordinary resiliency of the human body; the physical and mental effort required to come back; and the amazing team that supported that effort. Along the way I had to learn how to make the transition from giver to receiver, one of many transitions that became necessary in order to tread the road to survival.

Part three, "The Path," is a real-life exploration of the practices that can move us from disaster, physical pain, and emotional turmoil to a life of love, joy, and fulfillment. I know this path not just from study and the generous offerings of my wise teachers but because now I have walked it. I have fallen down face-first in dung. I have wiped away the blood, stitched up the wounds, and then taken the next step. When I have finished, I will have made a comeback that few would have believed possible.

Along the way I made new friends, some of whom are not as fortunate as I. Their prognoses say that they will not walk again or that they have little time left to live. There is no known cure for their condition, yet they have healed. Their stories have inspired me and I believe they will you as well.

I use the terms "heal" and "recovery" throughout. "Recovery" refers herein to the recuperative process from an illness or injury. "Healing" is often used for a similar purpose, but in a broader sense encompasses the view that we are all healing from something—a relationship, a loss, a fear, a *dis*ease, a *dis*comfort, our upbringing, and so much more. We will explore how complete healing is possible even when a cure is not.

ALL OF our lives are filled with subtle and major dukkha, and every gradation in between. The range of dukkha is so great that I often choose not to translate the word; I simply write "dukkha." Fortunately, in spite of what at times feels like dukkha's pervasive nature, it is only one aspect of the human experience, woven inextricably with life's exuberance, delights, triumphs, and pleasures. Also, fortunately, we know a great deal about the nature of dukkha. Consequently, we know how to practice and bring it to an end. That is *The Path.*

One aspect of communication involves the brain receiving information communicated by another and comparing it (instantaneously) to data it has previously stored. If there is comparable information we say, "I understand." If not, we can request an explanation, go to Google, or just let it go. When we attempt to share an experience that is far out of the norm, we often add adverbs such as "very," "extremely," or "awfully" to emphasize the uniqueness of our experience. But these additions can easily become repetitious and lose their meaning. This is a way of saying that I do not think I could possibly do justice to the profound nature of the experience outlined herein, so I have opted, for the most part, to let it speak for itself. I am confident, *extremely* confident, that you will get it.

It was not possible to bring this story to a conclusion because it is ongoing. It will, of course, come to an end, but even at that, my wish is that you carry on what I have offered here.

May you never know my experience, but may you benefit from it, and may all beings be happy, safe, and free from harm.

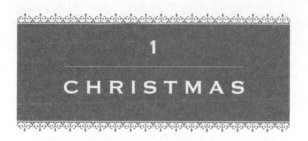

1

CHRISTMAS

MYANMAR

You Will Be All Right, Sir

On December 17, 2012, Susanna and I headed for Myanmar for an eighteen-day holiday. A week or so before we left, we saw pictures in the newspapers of President Obama and Secretary of State Hillary Clinton strolling through the magnificent Shwedagon Pagoda, which was one of our scheduled sites. Our already whetted appetites were now more so, and we were truly excited to go. Our first days, spent in Yangon, Bagan, and Mandalay, were delightful, with old and wonderful sights and literally thousands of ancient temples available for exploration. I had been studying the teachings of the Buddha and practicing Buddhist meditation since the nineties, so this trip had meaning on several levels for me. This essentially Buddhist land was beginning to take its place among our favorite destinations alongside our African safaris and excursions to India.

The evening of December 24, there was a big party at our hotel in Mandalay, with lots of people, food, music, and gaiety. Then, the morning of December 25, Christmas Day, we, along with some sixty-nine others, boarded Air Bagan flight number W9-011 for Heho Airport near Inle Lake, an area popular with tourists for its floating markets and unique method of fishing. (Fishermen stand with one leg in the boat, and the other in the water with a paddle tied to it. The paddle leg navigates the boat, leaving both hands free for fishing. This method apparently is not practiced anywhere else in the world.) There were some patchy low clouds outside as Susanna and I took seats a little more than halfway back on the left side of the plane. The twenty-five-minute flight left at 8:30 a.m. but never arrived at its destination. About a mile before the airport, we crashed.

At first I thought we just had a bad landing, so when Susanna said, "We've crashed," I thought she was overreacting. The plane went dark right away as we skidded, swirled, and bounced on the ground for five hundred or so feet. The cabin immediately began to fill with a dense, noxious, black smoke and the smell of jet fuel. We had torn through electrical wires as we came down and we could see outside our window that the plane was already ferociously on fire. We were in real and imminent danger.

The passengers started pushing toward the front of the plane. I held up my hands trying to calm them: "Easy, everyone, don't push, we'll all get out!" No one paid attention to me and I realized that they did not care what I was saying. I pulled Susanna in front of me intending that we also exit through the front of the plane. There was tremendous chaos and we were making no progress moving forward. Susanna turned back to me and said she did not think we could make it to the front exit, as she already could not breathe. We were near the emergency exit and although it was engulfed in roaring fire, we would have to jump out through the flames. With a nod of consent from Susanna, I gave her a push and out she plunged through the flaming doorway to the ground below. In retrospect I now realize that I had no idea what I was pushing her into or how far she would be jumping. There was no choice. It was all instinct. Jump or be scorched.

The open emergency door revealed that the plane was now seriously in flames, with the fire's searing arms blazing in every direction. As I made my move to follow Susanna, there was what proved to be a disastrous moment. My foot caught on something and I was stuck. I was not just surrounded by fire; I was now in it, and I could not move. I called out for help but no one responded. I was frightened. Perhaps more accurately, I was terrified. I could feel my heart pumping in my throat, yet at the same time I was fully present to the situation and quite calm. I worked quickly to release my leg and after a ferocious battle (which later Susanna told me took close to a minute), I freed myself. I also learned later that such was my effort to survive that I tore through the leather of my left shoe trying to free my leg. I jumped through the flames to the ground, but I was already severely injured.

There is a blank space in my memory from the time of struggling to free my leg to the time I was on the ground. I have no idea what happened in that time, but it must have been when I was most seriously burned. My trauma therapist refers to this type of memory loss as the work of the "benevolent brain." Susanna recalls those moments:

> Allan gave me a push and I leaped through the fire try-
> ing to land as far as I could from the plane, but my
> main concern was getting through the flames. I turned
> around and looked at the open door expecting to see
> Allan, but he didn't appear. I kept screaming his name
> again and again, but still no Allan. The heat of the fire
> was so intense and the smell of the burning fuel so nau-
> seating that I couldn't keep facing directly at the plane
> and ultimately had to move back some distance. I don't
> know how long it was, but it seemed interminable. I
> thought that perhaps Allan had found a way to get out
> the front of the plane because I saw other people sliding
> down the escape chute up there. As the time dragged
> endlessly on without my seeing Allan, I began to fear

that he was dead and I would never see him again. Then, suddenly, he appeared in the doorway. I screamed to him, "Jump! Jump!" and he did.

On the ground Susanna immediately grasped my arm and began to drag me away from the plane. I could not move my legs, but we gave it all we had until we could no longer move. She also did not know that she had suffered four broken vertebrae in the crash (not that anything would have stopped her from trying to carry me). A crowd was gathering and two teenage boys ran down and tried to help drag us up the slope where the plane had crashed. If I looked straight ahead, I saw the faces of the gathering spectators, who, as they stared at me, looked truly horrified. If I looked down, I saw large sheets of skin hanging from my hands and legs. That skin and those faces should have scared me, but I think I was simply too numb, too dazed, or too deeply in shock to realize the seriousness of my condition.

Kimberly and Marty, two Americans who were also passengers on the plane, escaped injury. They wrote an account of the event for family and friends that included the following:

A tall man had just jumped out of the wreckage and he was badly burned. A French-speaking passenger replaced one of the boys on the man's left, and Marty got on his right. The man was burned terribly, and unfortunately, it looked like a scene from a war movie. As they slowly walked, I tried to clear away the sharp dried rice stalks, since the man's clothing was mostly burned away, leaving him with no protection. He was obviously in shock, or fueled by adrenaline, because he said, "People say burns are painful, but I can't feel anything." Then he added, "I must look really bad. I can tell by the way people are looking at me." Marty wanted him to stay calm and said, "Nah, just a little sunburn." As we walked, the man told us that as he tried to jump from the plane his leg got caught on something.

We got away from the plane just in time and we heard four loud blasts as it exploded. It was more than a year later when I saw for the first time the "official photo" of the plane just before it exploded. The flames soared more than twenty feet high and the thick black smoke rose another thirty feet above that. It was a frightening sight and the realization that I had been inside that plane was numbing. The ground, a dried-up rice field, was rough and brambly and it slanted upward, making our trudge even more challenging. We were heading toward what seemed to be some sort of abandoned stone temple. We walked by passengers who had been on the plane with us, some hugging each other and others shedding tears of gratitude. Many of them escaped unharmed. There were other people lying on the ground with injuries of varying degrees of seriousness.

I heard that two people were killed in the accident. One was a motorcyclist who was in the field where the plane had crashed. It was months later that I learned that the other victim was Nwe Lin, our guide, who had been with us from the day we arrived in Myanmar a week earlier. Nwe Lin was in the seat right behind me. I lived. She died. The words of a song that I love come to mind: "Who can explain it? Who can tell you why? Fools give you reasons, wise men never try."[1] Buddhists account for these

---

[1] "Some Enchanted Evening," from Richard Rodgers and Oscar Hammerstein's *South Pacific.*

things by citing the "law of dependent origination," sometimes called "causes and conditions," or simply "conditionality." It means that nothing just happens. All phenomena are preceded by the causes and conditions that come together to make up each moment in time and space. While I believe this to be true, sometimes it is not enough to fill the emotional emptiness, the immense void that is left within me when there simply are no answers.

As Susanna and my two new friends dragged me up the hill through the throng of stunned spectators, a middle-aged woman with a serene face and an equanimous demeanor leaned out of the crowd and looked directly at me. When we were about an arm's length from each other, she quietly said to me, "You will be all right, sir." I never saw her before and I have never seen her since, but I cannot imagine that I will ever forget her. Surely there is no such thing as a stranger in this world. How many times in my moments of deepest despair have her words come back to me? "You will be all right, sir." Yes, my sweet nameless friend, I will. I will be all right. A moment of kindness, a compassionate smile, can not only uplift another being, it can save a life.

Since I was barely conscious, here is another account from Susanna:

There was the sound of a siren and we were loaded into an ambulance. This so-called ambulance was actually a panel truck that had a metal shelf attached to one wall. Allan was placed on that shelf, and I was laid down on the floor. The ride on the bumpy, hilly, curving "road" was often unbearable. I'm sure if I had not been so focused on Allan I would have vomited. The ride to the town of Taunggyi took about forty minutes, and the hospital was absolutely on a par with the ambulance. There was no electricity because when the plane crashed it tore down all the power lines. The room into which we were placed had two cots with no sheets and no pillows. There were no medical supplies, and no curtains on the window to shield us from the hot sun. There was a nonfunctioning sink hanging loosely from the wall, and like everything else in the room, it was filthy.

"You will be all right, sir" had been the prognosis of the woman on the hill. The doctor, however, did not agree. His professional opinion was that I could not possibly survive the injuries I had sustained. (This was spoken quietly to Susanna and I did not hear it.) Nevertheless, he did the "doctorly" thing. He hooked me up to an IV line and gave me a tetanus shot, even though Susanna told him I had had one three weeks earlier. That was the extent of my medical care in Myanmar since we never saw a doctor again. He assumed I was going to die and never returned.

There then appeared a woman named Miu Miu, a local bed-and-breakfast owner who was looking for one of her arriving guests whom she thought might have been on our flight. It turned out her guest had canceled at the last minute so Miu Miu said she was now there to help. She brought us sheets, pillowcases, water, and clothing. Susanna's pain was increasing and she was practically immobile.

Miu Miu took care of me. She gently washed me with bottled water and asked if she could cut off the pieces of burned clothing that were melted to my body, including my underwear. I said yes. As she did so, she quietly said to me, "Now I am

9

like your mother or your sister." She then dressed me in some clothing her husband had brought for me. I remember having a vague thought about feeling no discomfort with this woman removing all my clothing and washing every part of me. Nothing seemed to have any meaning; things were just happening.

Miu Miu was a gentle person and treated me with great kindness and respect. She was a Buddhist practitioner and would sometimes remind me, "You are not this body," words I had heard often through the years when I studied with the venerable Vietnamese monk, Thich Nhat Hanh. Knowing that we are much more than just a body is an important part of the teaching offered by the Buddha. Miu Miu's practical help was invaluable. She knew how to pay the nurses to get Susanna use of a bathroom and to buy some toilet paper. She got a wheelchair for Susanna since the pain she was now encountering made walking all but impossible.

SUSANNA: Allan was in very bad shape and rapidly getting worse. I had no concept about what burns did to the human body. It may be that I thought burns simply affected the surface of the body, the skin. Now I was learning that with burns of this depth and magnitude, the entire system is affected and Allan's body was shutting down. He was beginning to swell. His fingers, his legs, his face, all became puffy, with a gray-white color. His left eye closed completely, as his left side had suffered the worst burns.

No one spoke any English except Miu Miu. Then, as I was lying in the bed desperately trying to figure out some way to save Allan, a voice spoke gently in my ear, "We are here from the American embassy and we are going to help you." I was meeting Sai Oo, and his colleague Daniel Jacobs. They had been vacationing at Inle Lake with their wives. When they heard about the accident, they came to investigate and see if there were any Americans on board. They were told to go away; there were no Americans. Even so, they felt they wanted to see for themselves, just in case, so they came to the hospital in Taunggyi, where they found us.

The rest of the day was spent struggling to get us out of the hospital and taken to Bangkok. The officials insisted that all of the passengers had to be taken to Yangon. However, the other passengers were not as seriously injured, and the hospital in Yangon, while definitely better than Taunggyi, was not what Allan needed. There was an ambulance plane in Bangkok ready to come and get us, but the Burmese officials would not let the plane in over the border. The two American consuls kept negotiating, and finally the owner of Air Bagan, U Tay Za, agreed to send his private jet from Yangon to pick us up. It was not a medically equipped plane, but he was going to send a French national doctor to fly with us to Bangkok.

For Susanna, the day was filled with emotional dread and physical pain; my condition was rapidly declining and hers certainly was not getting any better. The wives of Sai Oo and Daniel Jacobs were invaluable. Daniel's wife was stationed in the embassy in Tokyo and was apparently quite helpful in facilitating our release. Toward evening we were taken by ambulance to a military base near the hospital. Susanna gave Miu Miu all the Burmese money she had, although she would not accept it until

Susanna insisted that she use it for her children. No amount of money could ever express our gratitude to this compassionate woman who had done so much for us.

We were put on a tiny helicopter, with Susanna and the pilot up front, and me lying on the floor behind them. A nurse from the hospital accompanied us. The consul drove ahead to the airport in Heho where U Tay Za had his private plane waiting for us. It was still light as the helicopter flew from Taunggyi to Heho. I did not see this, but months later Susanna recalled that it was extraordinarily beautiful as we flew over the green hilly landscape of Shan State in Myanmar.

> SUSANNA: The sun was setting as we got onto the plane at the airport. I was taken aback by the beauty of the sunset, and how ironic it was that I could experience it at the worst moments of my life. I was in a wheelchair with serious pain, and Allan was on a stretcher dying. There were many military personnel, and other officials around the airport, and I felt assaulted by their photographing and videoing Allan and me as we were moved to the plane.

BANGKOK

I was rarely awake during our three days in Bangkok, so here again is Susanna's account:

> An ambulance transported us from the airport. It was early evening as we sped to Bumrungrad Hospital, where we were admitted through the emergency room.

Allan was taken directly to the intensive care unit and I to a standard room. Again, there was a stark juxtaposition. It was an elegant hospital catering to foreign nationals, with such niceties as a fresh rose on the breakfast tray every morning, but it was not equipped to care for the severity of Allan's burns. That night a plastic surgeon/skin specialist worked on Allan and debrided much of the dead, burned tissue. The wounds were dressed with silver nitrate ointment and covered with bandages, but the doctor said that he must get to a burn unit as soon as possible. He told me that with burns it is essential that the patient be treated right away. Ideally, Allan would have been in a burn unit immediately after the accident.

The doctor also felt that Allan was so badly injured systemically that he needed to be stabilized before he could even be moved. He was the second doctor whose "official prognosis" was that Allan probably was going to die.

For three days in Bangkok Allan was stabilized, dressings changed around the clock, and since his veins were now closing down, a central line was inserted into his neck. He kept swelling and both of his eyes were now closed, although there were occasional times when he was awake and alert.

It became increasingly clear that if Allan had any chance to survive he needed to be moved as soon as possible to a real burn unit. We worked with a company called Global Rescue, which from that point on provided invaluable assistance with the complex transportation details. The big question was, where to go. New York was probably the best choice in terms of medical care, but it seemed unlikely that Allan could survive the lengthy flight. So we chose Singapore, which, we were assured, had the best burn unit in that part of the world.

Singapore General Hospital, however, demanded a deposit of two hundred and fifty thousand dollars before they would admit Allan. There would be no exceptions and no considerations—no pay, no stay. I was on the phone for many hours getting credit card limits increased, signing papers assuring that we could repay the money, and so forth. All of our efforts were in vain, until we were able to contact U Tay Za, who fronted the money to the Singapore hospital.

The air ambulance flight to Singapore took about five hours, which could only begin after Bumrungrad Hospital in Bangkok was satisfied that we had paid them in full.

SINGAPORE

When we arrived at Singapore's ultramodern hospital, they took me directly to the ICU burn unit. There was a lot of fuss made over us, the two new American patients. VIPs, airline representatives, and others all seemed to want to help. U Tay Za provided Susanna with an assistant named Melinda, a particularly sweet Burmese national living in Singapore. She was a Buddhist practitioner and a student of the Indian master, S. N. Goenka. She was incredibly efficient and quickly provided the things Susanna needed, such as clothing, toiletries, a phone, a computer, and a razor for me, all of which had been lost in the crash.

We then met Dr. Tan Bien Keem, whom we would soon come to know as a brilliant surgeon, a calming presence, a human being of extraordinary compassion, a healer, and in the truest, most meaningful way, a friend. BK, as he invited us to call him, was the first doctor to express the view that I would live. Naturally, we loved him. (Months after we left Singapore, he called us, and again his laughter and beautiful spirit lifted our hearts.)

Many decisions had to be made regarding how to keep me alive. Susanna signed documents granting permission to perform numerous surgeries and procedures. BK began grafting my burns by taking skin from my abdomen and thighs to transplant onto my head and hands. Later we would learn that these grafts were performed with a level of expertise that was little short of astonishing.

My legs were grafted with cadaver donor skin. While the grafts made of my own skin would become permanent, the cadaver skin would last only three weeks. It was still essential to use because skin apparently made the perfect bandage, and it protected me from infection, which is a major issue when dealing with burns. Further, BK explained, it would not have been advisable to take more skin from my body at that time, as it would have increased the possibilities for opportunistic infections. Besides which, I might not have survived such additional harvesting. Later, my back, abdomen, and thighs would be stripped of their skin for leg grafting and regrafting of my hands.

Dr. Tan was kind enough to summarize the medical procedures he performed on me:

SUMMARY FOR ALLAN LOKOS
AT SINGAPORE GENERAL HOSPITAL

Dec. 28, 2012
Admission to the Singapore General Hospital Burns Intensive Care Unit

1. Burn assessment

33% total body surface area burned, comprising deep dermal burns on both hands, partial thickness burns on the head, left buttock and a mixture of deep dermal and full thickness burns over lower limbs bilaterally.[2]

Operation #1—12/29/2012
Burns excision, split skin grafting (SSG) were performed on both hands. Cadaveric [human cadaver donor skin] and autologous [(your own skin] skin grafting were done to both legs [comprising 18% of total body surface area]. Burn excision and split skin grafting were done on the scalp on 12/29/12. Autologous skin was harvested from both thighs. VAC dressings [negative pressure dressing] were also applied to both lower limbs.

You were reviewed by hand surgeon, Dr. Andrew Chin on 1/1/13 and 1/2/13. His opinion was that your fingers were deeply burnt.

The ophthalmologist had also seen you and opined that the burn of the eyelid and face were superficial.

---

[2] The terms first-, second-, and third-degree burns are no longer used. What was a third-degree burn is now referred to as "full thickness burn."

Operation #2—1/2/2012
During the second operation, the previous cadaveric skin grafts were adherent and the autologous skin grafts over the right hand, left hand and scalp had taken well.

Operation #3—1/5/2012
You had a repeat dressing change and we found all the skin grafts had taken well, with a small unstable area over the left knee.

Operation #4—1/7/2012
Wound inspection showed skin graft took over the hand dorsum [upper side]. However, your fingertips remained necrotic [with dead tissue].

2. Microbiology
You remained afebrile [not feverish] throughout your hospital stay.

The Infectious Disease physician was consulted on 12/29/12 and his opinion was to continue intravenous antibiotics [tazocin and vancomycin].

3. Nutrition
Initially, feeding was through a nasogastric tube, and this was subsequently removed for better comfort as you were now able to eat and drink normally.

4. Rehabilitation
You underwent chest physiotherapy during your inpatient stay. You were taught deep breathing exercises, shoulder and elbow exercises, which helped in your recovery.

5. Hearing impairment

The otolaryngologist suggested audiogram after transfer out of the intensive care unit.

6. Transfer home

You were medically evacuated from SGH to New York–Presbyterian Hospital on 1/8/13.

I was heavily bandaged everywhere: hands, head, and legs. The extensive grafting of my legs required that they also be enclosed in pumps. These pumps sealed me off, as best as possible, from infection. They also continuously pumped out fluid and blood after the surgeries. BK explained to us that the healing of burns can be deceptive. It might look after a while as if the burns were healed, but beneath the surface the healing would go on for another year or two.

In several areas, my burns went all the way through to the tendons and bones. The index and middle fingers of my right hand had been quite severely damaged. Before one particular surgery, BK explained to Susanna that those two fingers might have to be amputated. She signed the necessary papers and then waited as BK and a hand surgeon entered the operating room. The damage was deep but when they were cutting away the dead tissue, fresh blood appeared. This told them that there was living tissue that could possibly regenerate. Before the surgery was over, they sent word to Susanna that the two fingers were saved. To date, those fingers still have necrotic tips,[3] but are essentially alive and

---

[3] The word "necrotic," in health circumstances, refers to the death of most or all of the cells in an organ or tissue due to disease, injury, or failure of the blood supply; it is a form of cell injury that results in the premature death of cells in living tissue.

well.[4] In the future they might need additional surgery to help them function better, but ten is ten and I am deeply grateful.

FROM SUSANNA: Dr. Tan discussed the amputation possibility with me the day before, but not with Allan. However, that evening while I was not there, the hand specialist went in to see Allan and told him about this possible amputation. When I came back to Allan's ICU bay we talked about it. Allan's understanding from the hand surgeon was that the decision to amputate the fingers had already been made. He was amazingly calm about it. He displayed, not for the first time, and certainly not for the last, an extraordinary equanimity about letting go into what he couldn't control. It was incredible and it helped me so much, as I struggled with the feelings that arose within me. I remember the night before the surgery thinking that if only those two fingers could be saved, then everything would be all right. I had no idea then of the difficulties and brushes with death that still awaited us.

God, grant me the serenity to accept the things I cannot change,
The courage to change the things I can,
And the wisdom to know the difference.

The Serenity Prayer, above,[5] became an integral part of Alcoholics Anonymous in 1941. The advice is straightforward:

---

[4] In January 2014, thirteen months after the accident, the last of the necrotic tissue came off.

[5] Credited to the American theologian Reinhold Niebuhr.

Investigate deeply to find the truth, and when it is best to relinquish that to which we are holding firmly, do so with as much grace as possible. When the current situation is unacceptable and can be changed, take action firmly and with perseverance. The Dalai Lama has said: "If there is a solution or a way out of the difficulty, you do not need to be overwhelmed by it. The appropriate action is to seek its solution. Then it is clearly more sensible to spend your energy focusing on the solution rather than worrying about the problem. Alternatively, if there is no solution, no possibility of resolution, then there is also no point in being worried about it, because you cannot do anything about it anyway."

I knew that Susanna was in a better position to make a wise decision for me than I was for myself, and I knew that we both trusted BK to look out for my best interests. The thought of losing two fingers was disturbing, to say the least, but my concerns were cushioned in the compassionate arms of equanimity. My years of mindfulness practice and an understanding of the necessity to relinquish what we must, served me well. Fortunately, the fingers were saved and there was no need for worry.

THE NURSES in Singapore were Asian, and as one would expect, most spoke only some rudimentary English. Mostly, they were caring and gentle. They probably had not tended to many Western men, because they often commented that I seemed so tall. When I had to be moved or turned, it took four of them to do so. They accomplished these maneuvers by each taking a corner of the sheet and lifting. I taught them to coordinate their moves by counting out loud. It came out something like, "Wuahn, tooo, trreee," then a great grunting tug, followed by considerable laughter (on their part, not necessarily mine).

Frankly, I think the nurses found this big Westerner enjoyable. One of them sobbed heavily when it was time for me to leave, which brought tears to my eyes as I had grown quite fond of her and her colleagues. Some came in on their day off so they could say goodbye to Susanna and me.

Their actions reminded me to never be too busy to be kind to others. If we are too busy to be kind, we are too busy.

A Tibetan monk came to visit me one day as he was passing through on his way back to Tibet. We spoke for quite a while about the dharma,[6] meditation, and what it is like to live life as a monk. It was wonderful to spend a couple of hours not focused on injuries, burns, and surgeries. Before he left he chanted and offered prayers. The Tibetans seem to me to be a particularly joyful people and I got a soothing lift from his visit.

I was reminded that in the Buddha's enumeration of the Seven Factors of Enlightenment, the fourth factor is *piti*, which means joy, rapture, or happiness. Although the monk left me feeling cheerful, I knew that no one is able to give to another the gift of happiness. Each of us has to cultivate it for him- or herself through reflection, effort, and even determination. Since happiness is a mental factor, it will not be found in external or material things, though sometimes they certainly may contribute for a short time and in a small way.

The same is true of unhappiness. Someone may speak to us in a way that we find rude or obnoxious, or a situation may be difficult and challenging, but the resultant feeling of unhappiness exists within ourselves and therefore can be changed only within ourselves. It often seems that if we could change the

---

[6] Dharma in its broadest sense encompasses all phenomena; cosmic law and order; truth. It is also the term used to refer to the teachings of the Buddha.

other person, or existing conditions, then we would be happy, but the reality remains that we can control only what goes on internally. This is a difficult concept to grasp because one's immediate response to a challenging situation is usually to try to change it, rather than look within where real change can actually be accomplished.

I have had ample opportunity every day since Christmas 2012 to be miserable due to physical pain and the inability to lead my normal life. I have learned that misery and bitterness are not my only options. It was difficult at first, and there are challenges every day, but I am also having fun and it is absolutely incredible to be alive. The healing process is hard work, but it offers an unparalled opportunity for a sense of accomplishment.

Contentment is a characteristic of a happy person. We might find it difficult to cultivate contentment, especially when dealing with physical pain or a life-threatening condition, but with mindfulness and skillful thinking, it can be done. Contentment is a dynamic state, not to be confused with passivity or apathy. Contentment arises from active awareness of what really matters. Thoughts and feelings are always arising, and challenging situations cause the mind to scurry even more quickly than usual. If we are to remain equanimous, we cannot yield to every desire and impulse that presents itself. Instead, we want to focus on developing contentment.

It can help to understand the difference between pleasure and happiness. The enjoyable feelings of pleasure are fleeting and ephemeral, while happiness, well developed, has the legs to go the distance. It is enduring.

Real happiness does not come through grasping or clinging but rather through relinquishing. We move in the right direction when we practice lovingkindness, morality, compassion, and wisdom. As eighteenth-century Scottish poet Robert Burns wrote in his epic poem "Tam o' Shanter":

> *Pleasures are like poppies spread:*
> *You seize the flower, its bloom is shed;*
> *Or like the snow fall on the river,*
> *A moment white—then melts forever.*

For the most part my mind was quite clear while in Singapore, although I experienced confusion and fear when awakening in the morning or coming back from a procedure. Susanna was always there in the early morning and after all surgeries, so that when I woke up I would see her face and hear her reassuring voice. I am told, however, that there were times when I was sleepy or medicated, and became confused. Apparently, using my heavily bandaged hands, I would try to pull off the bandages that were on my head. At one point, it seems that I needed restraints, with my hands tied to the bed rails in order that I not hurt myself. Frankly, I am glad I do not remember that.

The ever-thinking Susanna put her cell phone into a small plastic bag so that she could bring it into the sterile ICU environment. That made it possible for me to speak with my daughter, Samantha, and close friends. Sam was ecstatic to hear my voice and know that I was indeed alive. I then spoke with my friend and longtime teacher, Sharon Salzberg, who so delighted in the idea of being placed in a little baggie and brought into my room. Sharon's laughter, abundant and well-known to me, was heartening to hear.

BK was becoming ever more important in our lives, not just for his skill as a surgeon but for his extraordinary presence and compassion as a human being. Susanna recalls:

One morning—it was in fact New Year's Day—Dr. Tan came to see us, and after his medical update, surprised Allan by saying, "I watched you teaching on YouTube last night." Allan was astonished. It was on that day that Dr. Tan began his appointment as the Head of Plastic, Reconstructive and Aesthetic Surgery at Singapore General Hospital. As always, wherever he walked, other doctors, nurses, and staff followed closely, thirsting to learn. You could almost feel them leaning in so as not to miss a word he said. By now, he and Allan had established a wonderful relationship, and when Allan saw all of the *"Grey's Anatomy* wannabes" clustered around Dr. Tan, he said quietly, "Ah, when the master speaks, everyone listens." Dr. Tan paused for a moment, and then, with great respect and elegance, replied, "It is we who should be sitting at your feet." For Allan, to hear such a comment from someone he so admired was a deeply moving moment, and one that I am sure he will not soon forget.

Just before we left Singapore there was another beautiful moment between Dr. Tan and Allan. These two men faced each other and Dr. Tan took Allan's heavily bandaged hands in his and said, "I would like to read your books, but I have one request. Please promise that one day you will sign them for me." In a choked voice, Allan replied, "I promise."

BK gave us hope for the future. Through his surgical skills he began the process of rebuilding my injured body. He was also the first doctor to say that he believed I could return to full function. That alone would have won him our adoration. Before he spoke, he thought carefully and his words were well considered. We had complete faith in his prognosis. Later, I would come to understand that "full function" did not necessarily mean that my hands would be as they were before, but rather that I would be able to function. At first, I found the distinction disturbing, but I have now come to view it as rather miraculous. Whether it be fully functional as I was before, or a modified fully functional, BK's words changed everything for me. I felt uplifted and have not stopped working at my healing process ever since.

FROM SUSANNA: It was also helpful that Dr. Tan was realistic and not a Pollyanna. There was an area on the back of Allan's head that he felt would need grafting in the future because the burn was so deep, but eight months later there was barely some redness and slight scabs that were falling away. Allan's left ear was damaged. We learned that ears are quite vulnerable, not only because they protrude but also because they are mostly cartilage, with only a thin layer of skin on top. The skin had been burned away and Dr. Tan felt that the cartilage was too damaged to try to do anything surgically at that time. He thought that Allan might need some reconstructive surgery on the ear in the future, but a few months later Allan's ear totally healed with no treatment. None of us knew at the time that Allan was gifted with extraordinary survival and healing capabilities.

I have no idea if my survival and healing capabilities are any greater or lesser than the next person, but I believe that my years of meditation practice make it possible for me to be present to what is going on, without creating stress-producing scenarios. Research over the past several years strongly suggests that there is no illness or injury that is not exacerbated by stress. So it makes sense that keeping stress to a minimum allows the body's natural capabilities to function at their best.

IT APPEARED as if we would need to be in Singapore for several months, but after about seven days, BK suggested to Susanna that it was possible, and even advisable, to airlift me home to New York City as soon as possible. He explained to her that important grafting of hands, head, and legs had been done with my own skin, which would help protect me from infection. Further, and importantly, my vitals were stable. We were beginning to understand that the skin burns, as severe and extensive as they were, were only the external part of the damage that could be done to a body by burns. The entire mind/body mechanism could be affected. ICU psychoses, chronic pain, infection, and medication reactions all loomed as possible major issues.

In the meantime the accident was being well documented at home in the media. The January 5, 2013, edition of the *New York Post* reported:

NY POST
JANUARY 5, 2013

WEST SIDE GURU SURVIVES CRASH

Allan Lokos, world-renowned founder of the Community Meditation Center on the Upper West Side, was

among the survivors of a horrific plane crash in Myanmar on Christmas Day. . . . The plane carrying 71 passengers crash-landed in dense fog in a rice field and
burst into flames, killing two. . . . Lokos . . . has third-
degree burns on his legs, hands and head. He saved his
wife [Susanna Weiss] by pushing her out of the plane
through a fire-engulfed exit before he jumped through
the flames himself. . . .

The couple, who have been married for 20 years,
were rushed to a local hospital in a truck, where badly
burned Lokos, who is 6-foot-2 and 180 pounds, had to
lie on a metal shelf. The rural hospital had few supplies,
and locals donated sheets and pillowcases to comfort
the injured. . . .

Lokos, who has already had two surgeries, is still in
an ICU in Singapore, but is expected to return to New
York–Presbyterian Hospital on Monday. "He was amazingly strong, calm, very grounded and very centered. He
has been an amazing pillar of strength," said Weiss.
The Rev. Desmond Tutu has extended his prayers to the
couple.

New York radio station WNYC reported:

Members of the Community Meditation Center on the
Upper West Side met for the first time Sunday without
their leader, Allan Lokos, who survived a plane crash
with his wife in Myanmar last month. Lokos, a world-
renowned spiritual leader, sustained major burns to his
legs, arms and head. . . . His wife, Susanna Weiss,
suffered broken vertebrae. . . . Members of the center

gathered . . . waiting to hear updates on Lokos and his wife. . . . One of the board members . . . read a letter Weiss sent them: "Dear Sangha (community), Allan and I are in a strange land, with different languages, foreign customs and traditions. We've been in such difficult conditions and desperate circumstances with great physical, emotional and spiritual pain . . ."

Lokos . . . founded the center . . . [which] focuses on the practical aspects of Buddhism and meditation. . . . Speaking from Singapore last week, Weiss said that more than fifteen years of meditation has prepared them well for this. "The only way we've survived is being so in the present moment," she said. "For now we have to put the future aside because it's going to be a long, difficult road, and if you consider that, it would be just overwhelming."

On Sunday, Lokos's daughter Samantha Koppelman told the standing-room-only gathering at the Community Mediation Center that the first time she spoke to her father after the crash, he asked about how the Center was doing. "The most important gift you can give to my father and Susanna right now," she said, fighting back tears, "is to continue to show up here, and to bring your love, your prayers, your kindness, and your friendship that has overwhelmed me here from everyone."

NEW YORK

The news that we could, and in fact should, return home to New York was stunning. It even surprised the doctors at Johns Hopkins Hospital in the United States, who were monitoring the case closely. It seems that my body, though severely injured, remained incredibly resilient, for which I take no credit but am extremely grateful. It was BK's opinion that I was still drawing on my previous strength and this would be the best time to get me home. Otherwise, it would likely be months before another appropriate opportunity would present itself. Further, BK felt that I was as protected from infection as I could be in Singapore, but that conditions would be better in the United States. He also saw that Susanna could not continue on her own, with no family or friends, thousands of miles from home, with her own painful injuries, supporting me in all the ways I needed. It was important for Susanna and me to be home, but getting me back to New York was not going to be easy.

SUSANNA: I was frightened to authorize the thirty-hour air ambulance evacuation of Allan to New York City. It was yet another time when I felt Allan could die. However, once I had all of the details from Dr. Tan, and the time to carefully consider them, it seemed to me the right thing to do. It was in fact, in many ways, the only logical thing to do. Once I made the decision, I felt at ease; at least I think I did.

The arrangements were extremely complicated. Specialists who understood the pumps that kept Allan's grafted legs sealed and drained arranged for the proper batteries and chargers to keep them going through the long flight. The plane had to be reconfigured with outlets that could accommodate those chargers, coordinating Thai, Singapore, and US power systems, and that was just one of many technical issues.

The small jet would have to stop at least five times

to refuel and change crews. There was room on board for the pilot, the copilot, a doctor, one other medical person, and Allan. There was no room for me. It was unbearable to realize that I had to let Allan make this flight without me. There was some small comfort in the fact that he would be sedated and closely monitored throughout the flight.

Every time the flight was organized, with all of its complex details, it would then all fall apart when Singapore would not issue a permit for the origination of the flight. I was booked on an eighteen-hour commercial flight from Singapore to New York that would leave at about the same time as Allan's flight. I had to keep changing my flight because I refused to leave until Allan's plane was actually in the air. Ultimately, Allan had to be driven by ambulance to Malaysia for his flight, as Singapore never did come through with the proper permits.

My plane arrived in New York the evening of January 8. Our daughter, Samantha, met me at the airport and she couldn't stop touching me, holding me, and crying on me.

Susanna and I soon found that friends who saw us for the first time after the accident would usually burst into tears and need to touch us. I felt particularly moved by one of our first friends who visited me in the New York hospital. As I rolled toward her in my wheelchair, she clutched her heart and, with moist eyes and a hushed voice, could only say, "Oh my God. Oh my God. Oh my God."

SUSANNA CONTINUES: Through the night, Samantha and I stayed in touch with Global Rescue, the company that arranged the medevac flight. Sam and I would get updates on our cell phones about where the flight was, and how Allan was doing. As promised, he was sedated throughout the whole flight and carefully monitored by the doctors on board.

Early in the morning of January 9, my plane arrived at Teterboro Airport, about twelve miles from Midtown Manhattan. Susanna was allowed to come out onto the tarmac so she could greet me, tell me where I was, and assure me that everything was all right. I doubt that I understood much of anything she was saying, but it must have felt good to her. I was transported by ambulance, with siren blaring, to the burn unit of New York–Presbyterian Hospital, where Susanna was soon again at my side.

The ensuing scene was chaotic, with a dozen or more medical people buzzing around me. Everyone seemed to be in "emergency mode," which is, perhaps, the way they viewed the situation. I am sure their preference would have been to treat me two weeks earlier when the burns first occurred. As mentioned, with serious burns, immediate treatment is highly advantageous. My burns were now fifteen days old.

The frenetic scene reminded me of what happens so often at a more joyous occasion, a wedding day. There is a great deal of hustling and bustling, with the caterer checking with the bride as to whether these are the right size shrimp, the hairdresser tucking in a loose end, the makeup artist patting away a bead of perspiration, and the photographer yelling, "Look this way!" All are well intentioned; all want to do their job well; all want to serve the couple honorably. Yet the poor bride finds herself being driven to distraction. Somehow, I managed to remain calm. The fact that I was inordinately drugged probably helped.

SUSANNA RECALLS: There was a not-so-subtle, derogatory tone from some of the staff regarding the treatment Allan had received in Singapore. One male head nurse said to me, "You'll find that we do things differently here in New York. For example, we don't use xenografts here." I asked what that meant and he said it is when animal skin is grafted onto a human. I told him that was not done to Allan. He replied, "Well, that's what we were told, that he had pig skin grafted onto him," and he walked away.

While that seemed an unskillful comment, it made it even more satisfying when, later on, one of America's most respected surgeons, Dr. Roger Yurt, while inspecting Allan's right hand, asked, "Are you sure this was grafted? It doesn't show."

Dr. Yurt and Allan got along well, possibly because they are both funny guys. One time Allan asked the good doctor if all of his grandchildren's tuition was secured, and if not, perhaps the two of them could find another surgery to perform on Allan.

Allan was brought into "the tank," where they debride the burns by scraping off the dead tissue. What is beneath is then scrubbed away until they get down to fresh, bleeding, live tissue. While this is an important step in burn care, and cause to rejoice when there is live tissue underneath, it is a horrible experience for the patient, and unfortunately Allan had to go through it many times.

It was extremely regrettable that the first time in the tank was egregiously mishandled. In order to help Allan cope with the extreme pain of the procedure, they readied him by giving him ketamine, a hallucinogenic drug known on the street as "Vitamin K." However, the preparation was awful. He was rushed into the tank with about eight people working on him at once, and there was loud rock music playing. As Allan was rolled in, one of the staff said to him, "Hey, how do you like our music?" Allan told me he said, "Actually, I am a classical musician and I prefer something quieter." The staff member said, "Oh, come on, you'll love this, let's get with it." The bright lights, the metal table, the pain, the music, the many people hovering around him all at once, caused Allan to have a classic hallucinogenic "bad trip."

When he came back to the room, he described it to me and said that he had been sure he was dying. He also felt that he was glad he was dying because the "trip" was so awful, that the only way he could find peace would be in death. He remembered the Tibetan teachings of traveling through the bardo into death.[7] What was happening to him felt like the experience of death as described in great detail by Sogyal Rinpoche in *The Tibetan Book of Living and Dying*.

As best I can describe this unfortunate experience, my entire field of vision was filled with a gigantic ceramic tile, which

---

[7] The Tibetan word "bardo" describes an intermediate or transitional state.

was, except for the size, similar to a kitchen or bathroom tile. Within the tile were many smaller tiles, brightly painted with various designs. The giant tile began to spin and the spinning became faster and faster. With that, the already loud rock music became louder and louder. Things became so fast and so loud that I became desperate for it to stop, but it would not. I do not remember how long this went on, but it seemed endless. When it finally ended, I was limp and exhausted.

Back in my ICU bay, I asked to speak with the doctor, and to his credit, he apologized, acknowledging that such an experience should never have happened and that he would see that it never happened to me again. I appreciated what he said. Nevertheless, what happened had already happened, and I had to deal with it. Through my meditative practice, I have learned how to be aware of what is going on in my mind, and then, if necessary, gently release what might be causing stress or unhappiness. It took a couple of days for me to be free of this unfortunate incident.

BACK TO SUSANNA: By then it was late in our first day back in New York. We were distraught, discouraged, and exhausted. We asked each other, "What have we done?" We thought we were in the best place in the world to save a life, but instead it seemed as if we had descended into hell. As Allan lay there, wrapped almost entirely in white bandages, we cried with each other. We could not touch or hold each other, which both of us desperately needed.

I stepped out of the room to consult with the doctor. As he spoke with me he painted a grim picture. He told me how extensive and deep the burns were and how at risk Allan was for all sorts of serious medical issues. He ended his report by telling me that there was still a real possibility that Allan would not make it. I was stunned. Allan had survived the ordeals of the crash in Myanmar, the frustrations of Bangkok, the surgeries in Singapore, and several strenuous medevac flights. Now to be told that he still might not make it was simply too much to bear.

THE TWO great wings of Buddhist teachings are "compassion" and "wisdom." Both need to be cultivated and practiced if we are going to fly in the rarified air of awakening. To truly understand and practice compassion, we must start with ourselves. We may be reluctant to feel our own suffering because it can be accompanied by self-blame and regret. Yet to be in the world as a compassionate being, we must practice self-compassion. Without compassion for self, I do not believe that Susanna or I would have survived this ordeal. Compassion is a state of mind that is open and inclusive. It allows us to meet our suffering more directly. We see that we are not alone; everyone goes through difficult, even unbearable times. That oneness is the ground of compassion. It is our common humanity.

THE DAYS that followed were filled with all sorts of medical procedures and a sense of mental and emotional numbness. A great deal of time went to changing my dressings, which had to be done twice a day. Every bandage was removed from my hands, legs, head, and face. They were then re-dressed and re-bandaged. The process took about two hours each time. Even with the most gentle of nurses, it was painful and debilitating.

I do not remember how many surgeries, grafts, and other

procedures were performed during those days, but there were quite a few. My legs, which had suffered deep burns, were originally grafted in Singapore with donor cadaver skin. Such skin lasts no more than three weeks and is used primarily in emergencies. Now the doctors needed my own skin to create permanent grafts. It was taken from my back, abdomen, and inner thighs. They needed a lot of skin, since the leg burns were extensive. They attached the grafted skin with hundreds of surgical staples, which were later removed.

Dr. Yurt was kind enough to summarize the medical care I received at New York–Presbyterian Hospital. It offers a view of the extent of my injuries.

*Please note: This medical summary
contains graphic descriptions of surgical procedures.*

January 9, 2013: Arrival. Open wounds and weight loss [~7%, 185 to 160 lbs.]

January 11, 2013: OPERATION #1
Pre-operative diagnosis: 32% total body surface area burns, all full thickness [third-degree] on both thighs and both lower legs.

Procedure: Tangential excision [sequential removal of layers of burn wound with specialized knives until all dead tissue is removed] and split thickness allograft of both thighs and both lower legs.[8] Anesthesia: general.

---

[8] An allograft is a graft made of tissue taken from a donor, usually a cadaver, of the same species as, but with a different genetic makeup from, the recipient, such as a tissue transplant between two humans. An "autograft" is skin taken from the patient. An "eschar" is a slough, or piece of dead tissue, that is cast off from the surface of the skin, often after a burn injury.

Findings: There was a mixture of open wound [raw red areas], residual eschar [dead skin] and allograft and autografted wounds. The excised areas were deep partial [deep second degree] and full thickness [third degree— all the way through the skin].

After the induction of general anesthesia you were prepped and draped in a sterile manner. The wounds were excised with Humby[9] and Goulian knives.

Allograft [cadaver skin] was obtained from The New York Firefighters Skin Bank and was approximated to the wound edges with staples. Adjacent sections of graft were approximated with Weck clips.

Your knees and feet were immobilized with splints that stayed on for three days. The excised and grafted area was 4181 square centimeters.

Blood loss was 800 cc and you received two units of packed red blood cells.

January 18, 2013: OPERATION # 2
Pre-operative diagnosis: 32% total body surface area burned, all full thickness (3rd degree) on both thighs and both lower legs.

Procedure: Tangential excision and split thickness autograft (your own skin) of both thighs and both lower legs. Anesthesia: general.

---

[9] A Humby is a large knife with a 10-inch blade and an adjustment to change the thickness of tissue that is removed. A Goulian is a shorter knife composed of a razor blade like a barber's razor that is about three inches long and can be set to remove 8/1000 to 30/1000 of an inch of tissue.

You had two grafting procedures in Singapore and your legs were excised and allografted last week. You were now ready for the second stage autografting of these areas.

Findings: There was a mixture of open wound, residual eschar and allograft and autografted wounds. The excised areas were deep partial and full thickness.

After the induction of general anesthesia, you were turned to the prone position, and prepped and draped in a sterile manner. Autograft skin was harvested with a Zimmer Dermatome machine.[10]

You were turned to the supine position and the wounds were excised with Goulian knives. The autograft was approximated to the wound edges with staples. Adjacent sections of graft were approximated with Weck clips.

Your knees and feet were immobilized with splints.

Blood loss was 700 cc and you received two units of packed red blood cells.

January 24, 2013: *Klebsiella*[11] bacteria found in the blood; probably came from your wounds; treated with meropenem.

January 25, 2013: Urinary tract infection treated with meropenem.

---

[10] Zimmer Dermatome is a nitrogen pressure-driven machine that removes a thin layer of skin at a thickness of 10/1000 of an inch after the subdermal injection of PlasmaLyte (a balanced salt solution that is injected under the skin to make it smooth and tight).

[11] *Klebsiella* organisms can lead to numerous diseases, specifically sepsis, pneumonia, urinary tract infections, and soft tissue infections. Meropenem is a broad-spectrum antibiotic used to treat a wide variety of infections.

January 28, 2013: OPERATION # 3

Pre-operative diagnosis: 32% total body surface area burn with full thickness [third degree] on both hands and left lower leg. There is instability of PIP joint [proximal interphalangeal; this is the middle joint of the finger] second finger of right hand.

Post-operative diagnosis: Same, plus instability of PIP joint of fifth finger on left hand.

Procedure: Tangential excision and split thickness autograft of both hands and the lower leg and temporary arthrodesis of the PIPs of right second and left fifth fingers.[12] Anesthesia: general.

You were now ready for autografting of open areas on your hands and left leg.

After the induction of general anesthesia, you were prepped and draped in a sterile manner. The wounds were excised with Goulian knives.

Autograft skin was harvested with a Zimmer Dermatome after the subdermal injection of PlasmaLyte. The autograft was approximated to the wound edges with staples.

0.045 Kirschner wires were passed through the PIP joints of the second right finger and the fifth left finger with a power drill.

The excised and grafted area was 156 square centimeters including 151 on the hands and 5 on the leg.

---

[12] "Arthrodesis" is the surgical joining of a joint by a procedure designed to accomplish fusion of the joint surfaces by promoting the proliferation of bone cells.

Blood loss was 100 cc and you received two units of packed red blood cells. There were no complications except that the urine in the Foley catheter was blood-tinged after moving the patient to the OR table. The catheter was removed and replaced under sterile conditions. I discussed this with your wife at the end of the procedure.

January 30, 2013: Cramps and diarrhea; tube feeding changed.

Early in December 2013, I had this e-mail exchange with Dr. Yurt:

LOKOS: *Based on my injuries that you saw, is it possible for you to estimate how long I might have been exposed to the fire? There is a blank spot in my memory that we would like to fill in as part of my psychotherapy.*
YURT: *It is difficult to tell. The extent of burn injury is dependent on the intensity of the heat and the duration of exposure. Best guess in your case would be less than a minute, especially if clothes caught fire, and possibly a few seconds if you were engulfed in flames.*

Having no medical background, I found this whole process quite miraculous, which was a lot better than focusing on my own discomfort. That attitude became more useful as it turned out that my hands also had to be regrafted. The burns were deep in places, as mentioned previously, going all the way down to the tendons and bone. So there I was in bed with bulky splints and dressings on both hands and legs. Since so much skin had been taken from my back, it was now difficult to find a comfortable position in which to rest.

Then there was the matter of apnea, which caused me to often wake up with a start.[13] Susanna stayed at my bedside for lengthy periods, and when I would wake up in this startled way, she would remind me of where I was and that I was okay. Many medications and most nutrition coming through a nasogastric tube led to periods of sharp abdominal pains. Because of the ongoing pain caused by the burns, this additional pain seemed particularly unwelcome. Nevertheless, it was all somehow manageable, perhaps because acceptance seemed to be the only real option.

I began having a difficult time getting through the night, which may have been a form of ICU psychosis.[14] The stress on my family members steadily increased. Even though we hired a nighttime nurse, I apparently was comfortable at night only when Susanna or Samantha was with me. Susanna spent twelve to fourteen hours with me each day, and on most days Samantha, with the support of her husband and little four-year-old, was with me for a few additional hours. Sam also took on the responsibility of providing more appealing food than the hospital offered. It was not all that difficult to outdo the hospital standard and she did a terrific job. There is something about good food that can brighten the darkest moments.

Even with healthier food now coming into me, I was weak

---

[13] "Apnea" is a suspension of breathing, which can occur as a consequence of neurological disease or trauma.

[14] ICU psychosis is a disorder in which patients in an intensive care unit experience anxiety and/or paranoia, hear voices, see things that are not there, become disoriented or agitated, and so forth.

and vulnerable. At various times and for innumerable reasons I had tubes coming out of every part of me: catheters, rectal tubes, nasal tubes, and tubes in places I did not even know there were openings.

The skin is the body's largest organ and protects us from many kinds of bacteria and illnesses. Burns, by their very nature, destroy skin tissue, leaving the patient vulnerable to infection and making infections from burns a major medical concern. These infections often lead to the death of the patient. I had many open areas on my body where skin had been taken for grafts.

An increasing problem in hospitals is that they now must deal more and more with strong antibiotic-resistant bacteria, a situation that has most likely been exacerbated by our overuse of antibiotics. Now, as if there was not enough with which to deal, there arose within me a new and serious problem. As the doctors had feared, I developed sepsis, a life-threatening infection.[15] The powerful antibiotics used to fight the sepsis caused uncomfortable side effects, and the drugs were taking their toll on my overall condition. I became weaker than ever. Fortunately, the sepsis was defeated within a few days, which allowed the doctors to stop the antibiotics, and I slowly regained a bit of strength.

There was some concern that I might have suffered permanent lung damage. In Bangkok, I was expelling large amounts of thick, black mucus. In Singapore, I was given daily breathing treatments through the oxygen mask that I was wearing. My faint memory of this is that it was quite unpleasant. Now, in

---

[15] Sepsis is a potentially deadly condition characterized by an entire body inflammation caused by severe infection. It kills millions of people around the world each year.

New York, it was determined that my lungs were clear and there was no damage. In the truest sense, I could breathe more easily.

THERE WAS a period when apparently I would slip in and out of delirium. Thankfully, Susanna reported, I was usually quite cheerful in my delusory state. She told me that I went back to my days as a professional singer/actor and began exuberantly declaiming great monologues. Evidently, sometimes I made them up; other times I offered the classics. One of my favorites was from *Man of La Mancha* and it seems I offered it frequently and with great fervor: "What is illness to the body of a knight-errant, what matter wounds? For each time he falls, he shall rise again, and woe to the wicked." It is such a dauntless and romantic exclamation. I love it. Although I was not fighting windmills, like the heroic Don Quixote, I was wounded and delusional. The reviews from staff and fellow patients were that I had a good voice. Not bad for someone whose professional career began all the way back when I was in the original Broadway production of *Oliver!* How embarrassing my vocal bellowings seem now but, if I'm lucky, I will never see that hospital staff or any of the other patients again.

I was told that in another moment of delirium, Susanna offered me some water. I responded, "No, I must not drink this. His Holiness needs it." Seemingly, I was concerned about the Dalai Lama and somehow felt that he might be particularly thirsty. Susanna assured me that His Holiness was fine and well attended and that it was okay for me to drink the water. After a moment of thought, my next concern was, "But what about the poor Tibetan people?" Susanna smiled broadly and convinced me that the Tibetan people would be fine if I drank the water, and so I did.

Add to this, that near the end of my stay at New York–Presbyterian Hospital, one of the doctors told Susanna she was concerned that I might have suffered brain damage due to anoxia while I was trapped in the fire.[16] Her assessment, it seems, was caused by my temporary inability to concentrate or remember things. Her diagnosis turned out to be incorrect and all my mental faculties ultimately returned. As one might easily imagine, the anguish suffered by Susanna and Samantha by this hasty and incorrect evaluation was unendurable. With all they had been through, starting with saving my life and including suffering through my delusional states, plus the fear that I might never be myself again, made this medical error a deeply traumatic experience.

There was, in fact, no shortage of traumatic experiences. Because I had so many surgeries and so many staples were used to close them, I suppose it was inevitable that one or two would be overlooked and not removed. One of my physical therapists noticed that two staples appeared to remain in my left pinky. She could feel them even though they were now beneath the surface, where skin had grown over them. We went to the surgeon's office and he brought in a big, burly colleague to remove the well-ensconced little steel devils. As this linebacker tugged and grunted, I came as close as I ever have to fainting. The bloody staples were finally extricated and fell to the floor, but somehow, I did not.

On a sweeter note, during the time when my hands were completely bandaged, and because of the high risk of infection, Susanna and I were not really able to touch each other. Anyone, including Susanna, entering my ICU bay was required to wear

---

[16] Anoxia is an absence or deficiency of oxygen.

protective gowns, masks, foot coverings, and gloves. The first time we were able to embrace was near the end of my two-month hospitalization. Susanna put her head down on my chest and I wrapped my arms around her. The tears that flowed were tears of unalloyed joy.

ONE MORNING near the end of my New York hospital stay, a doctor entered my room and introduced himself as part of the psychiatric staff. He said he had heard that I had been quite emotional during my stay. I told him that in spite of being an American male in our John Wayne–like rough-and-tumble society, I felt comfortable allowing my tears to be seen if something struck me as particularly joyful or overwhelmingly sad. I acknowledged that during my hospital stay there were numerous moments of deep sadness, as well as a few of incredible joy. My own view was that under the circumstances, there were not an inordinate number of such moments, and consequently my output of emotion was not out of proportion. Nevertheless, the doctor strongly recommended that I take a particular, "extremely mild" medication. Against my better judgment, and undoubtedly because I was in no condition to argue, I agreed.

About a week after leaving the hospital, I asked my primary physician, for whom I have the utmost respect, about my coming off that medication. He said it would be fine to do so, but I had to taper off slowly. In fact, it would require a full month to safely discontinue use of this "extremely mild" medication. I am not sure if I laugh more and cry less now than I did back then, but I do believe that allowing tears to flow naturally can be therapeutic. Suppressing our feelings, whether through conscious effort or the use of chemicals, has the potential to be harmful. A physician friend told me that she felt our use of prescription drugs was of epidemic proportions. Then again, we do not want to be denied the benefits of modern medicine. Therefore, the guidance of a competent and experienced psychopharmacologist can be invaluable.

There were times when my delusions were not so cheerful and, therefore, not as easy for my loved ones to handle. Sometimes I must have been confused and not understood where I was or what was going on. I often thought I had something in my hands and tried to give it to Susanna or Samantha. I would ask them to take care of it and make sure it would be safe. I wonder if I did this because I actually had things in my hands—splints and bandages. While this sounds harmless enough, in my disturbed mental state, this hand business became more frequent and I became more insistent. All of my systems and organs, including my mind, were suffering from the burns, and my poor loved ones had no idea when, or if, I would recover.

There were extraordinarily wonderful nurses who offered their considerable skills, caring, and experience. There were indifferent nurses who were, well, indifferent. There were also one or two who simply seemed incompetent. Susanna struggled with her issues about challenging authority and asked to have these nurses removed from my case. She feared that there might be repercussions in the form of other staff not providing me with good care, but to everyone's credit, that did not happen.

ONE MORNING Susanna entered my room and found me shaking violently. I was dealing with severe chills. I had no fever but my heart was racing. The nurse on duty administered IV doses of heart medication, but to no avail. It took a while, but it was ultimately Susanna and me, using our meditative skills, that brought my heart rate under control. We would soon find out that this was the beginning of my sepsis infection.

> SUSANNA REMEMBERS THINKING: After all this time, and all from which I had saved Allan, now he was going to die. Yet I was actually calm, perhaps from having been through this several times before. Now, in retrospect, I think I was calm through this terribly trying period because I was functioning in survival mode. Like the mother who can lift a car to save her child's life, I had to do impossible things again and again. My feelings went deep and I certainly wasn't numb, but there was no time for feelings while Allan was in crisis.

The days began to resemble one another, long, tiring, and filled with ever-emerging concerns. My medical needs seemed endless, and not only was there no progress, but things appeared to be going downhill. Most of the time I had no real sense of who I was or where I was.

Ultimately, however, small improvements began to happen. Smaller bandages were now being used on my hands and I felt less restricted. As I healed from the sepsis infection, I began to have greater mental clarity. I was extremely weak from lying in bed for so long as well as from the major trauma I had experienced. I was told that I was looking better and better but that healing would take a long time, probably around two years.

Physical therapists began to work with me every day. At first they just moved my fingers and hands, and then, after several days, they had me stand. It was then that I learned the shocking reality that I no longer knew how to walk; or perhaps I knew how, but my muscles were not strong enough to carry out the instructions from my brain. The first time I tried to stand up, it took three of those determined therapists to help me get out of bed. Their instructions as to how to stand and walk were clear, but somehow they did not translate into my being able to move. I felt like a bad student, a failure, but I knew I had to continue the effort because it was important to me to walk if I possibly could.

These sessions were long, arduous, and scary, but I kept reminding myself that I could do this. I could walk. I believe that, once or twice, I even had something akin to a panic attack. When that happened, the therapists calmly took me back to my room so I could sit or lie down, but I never let a session end that way. I would ask that they let me try it once more, and they always obliged.

The first time I took more than a couple of steps and walked out into the hallway, the doctors and nurses who were on duty saw me and gave me a big hand. By then I had been a patient for a long time, and for better or worse, I was well-known to the staff. It was not a standing ovation on Broadway, but it sure felt good. Today, I walk confidently and comfortably and even manage stairs without too much effort.

The fire with which I had done battle came at me primarily from my left side. Therefore, my burns were mostly on my left, and on the left side of my right limbs. One painful issue resulted from the flames coming so close to my left eye. At first it was puzzling, but the doctors finally concluded that the cornea was drying out. My eyes were not damaged by the fire, but due to scarring, my left eye was not closing all the way, even when I was asleep. So we had to keep the eye constantly lubricated, an hourly chore taken on by Susanna and Samantha. For many months we have been using silicone-impregnated strips around the eye, with the hope that eventually it will be able to close completely. Silicone, it turns out, helps to flatten and soften scars.

LIKE SO MANY of us, I often feel critical of our health care system, but there is no question that there are some extraordinary doctors practicing within the system. These are men and women with remarkable skills and extraordinary compassion. My primary care physician came to visit me several evenings a week at the end of his long and busy days. No matter what my mood at the time, it turned joyful whenever Mike appeared. He visited not just as a doctor but also as a friend and healer.

Fred is another doctor/friend, a cardiologist whose visits were more social than medical, although he was always in touch with my heart's condition. It was monitored electronically both at the nurses' station and at his office. He referred to what was going on within me as "an amazing event." He saw it as a classic struggle between the enormity of the disaster I had experienced and myself—the calamity versus the meditator, the teacher of patience. This seemed to move Fred deeply and he spoke about it often when he visited.

Humankind being as humankind is, not all doctors are the same. Mike, Fred, and BK are examples of doctors who are compassionate and caring. On the other end of the spectrum, in May 2013, I learned that I had a bladder stone that probably formed as a result of all the catheterization while in the hospital. The surgeon who removed the stone seemed a decent fellow, but after the surgery, he didn't return my calls or those from my pharmacy. When I finally reached him and had my questions perfunctorily answered, I mentioned that I was surprised that I never heard from him after the surgery as a courtesy to see how I was feeling. He sounded astonished. "I have been doing this for ten years," he said, "and I have never called a patient after surgery."

The good news is that he is young and perhaps will learn. The bad news is that this may be "the new doctoring."

Q. What do you call the person who finishes last in their class in medical school?

A. "Doctor."

Now, each day, one by one, nurses were withdrawing tubes and wires from my various orifices, and I was looking less and less like a weird sea creature. I was able to sit up for longer periods and to take longer walks in the hallway, often with very little support. Talk began to arise about transferring me out of my ICU bay and into rehab, another wing of that mammoth hospital complex. So it came to be that one bright winter morning, I was moved into an actual hospital room with such luxuries as my own shower and a chair. Several times each day I would have physical and occupational (hand) therapy sessions. At first, an aide took me to them in a wheelchair, but before too long I was walking to those sessions unassisted—gingerly, but nevertheless unassisted.

Burn dressings now were to be changed just once a day, but in the rehab wing, the nurses were not as familiar with the long and elaborate process. Back in ICU, Susanna had often assisted the nurses and now she was actually guiding the rehab nurses. Unfortunately, as the nurses learned how competent Susanna was, they began to leave the changing of burn dressings entirely to her. She was wise enough to ask for help, since for her this bandaging process was difficult and upsetting. Some of the trained ICU nurses eventually came and taught the rehab nurses. This was yet another instance when Susanna had to fight for what was best for me.

In a hospital everyone needs an advocate. I once asked one of the nurses how patients who were as seriously injured as I was managed if they did not have an advocate, or at least some kind of family support. The nurse replied, "They usually die."

As it became evident that my release date was drawing near, the dream of finally going home was becoming an exciting yet unsettling reality. Then, over the next several days, I had the most peculiar experience. I have lived in my New York apartment for more than forty years, yet as I tried to envision it, I could not. I could not see any of it. I could not see the living room, the bedrooms, the kitchen, none of it. I tried and tried because it seemed incomprehensible that I could not conjure up even one accurate view of something with which I was so familiar. For several nights, I had a recurring dream that took place in what I believed was supposed to be my apartment. Not only did it not look familiar, but it was being inhabited by a number of friends who were running some sort of illegal business activity there. I asked one of the staff psychiatrists what she thought this was about, and she said she had no idea. She advised me not to worry about it because I would see my home soon enough.

HOME,
(MOSTLY) SWEET HOME

When the day finally arrived, we loaded up Samantha and her husband Sean's car with the many gifts, mail, and assorted health care necessities that we had accumulated over the past two months. As I stepped from the wheelchair into the car,

I thought about what an incredible moment it was. I had not stood on anything but hospital floors for so long. I was surprised that we could fit my grin inside the car. We drove downtown and I looked at the city with wonder; it was as if I was seeing this magnificent megalopolis for the first time. New York, my hometown and residence for all my life, sparkled with the winter chill and never looked so glorious.

As we entered the lobby of our Upper West Side building, members of the building's modest staff greeted us. The morning doorman, who I had always believed did not particularly like me, tearfully embraced me. There was a big "Welcome Home" sign hung on our apartment door, the very door that only an hour earlier I could not envision.

My welcome home also included learning that my hands were too weak to turn the key in the front door. Susanna opened it and stepped aside so I could walk in first. Recall was instantaneous. I immediately remembered every detail but, more important, it now seemed to me the most beautiful place on earth. I reverently removed my shoes and walked slowly through each room, savoring every table and chair, every pot and pan, our bed, and my desk, oh, my desk, where I had spent some of the most creative hours of my life. Our home was more stunningly elegant than I could ever have imagined. It was indeed a superb homecoming.

I WILL ADMIT to being something of a "neat freak." I believe the term is "anal retentive." I like to know where things are and I rationalize my little idiosyncrasy by saying that I do not have to waste time looking for a particular book, CD, shirt, or other such object. (Albert Einstein reputedly had seven suits, each of which was exactly the same as the others. He said that he did this so he would not have to waste time deciding what to wear.) I quickly realized that my highly organized self would need to step aside while others handled, mishandled, and misplaced my various and sundry worldly thingamabobs. It was not a terribly difficult adjustment to make once I accepted that, at least for a while, my home was going to be a "home/hospital," and hospitals can have many people in and out all day long.

After a few minutes, Sam and Sean came up with bags and boxes full of the vast array of paraphernalia that we had collected during my hospital stay. There were gifts of Buddhist images and statuary; an endless assortment of cards, letters, and other forms of good wishes; flowers; plants; and medical supplies. It was a disruptive yet heartwarming sight for the neat freak.

The four of us settled into Susanna's studio where our recumbent exercise bike happens to unobtrusively reside. Almost without realizing it, I found myself on the bike pedaling away. My little family unit stopped what they were doing and stared at me with widened eyes. After I had barely survived a plane crash on the other end of the earth, followed by more than two months of hospitalization, I guess that the lure of physical movement was irresistible. The seduction lasted only about five minutes, which, considering everything, was pretty darn good. I then sat and rejoined the welcoming celebration.

That night, together again in our own bed, Susanna and I spoke about how extraordinary, indeed how unbelievably miraculous it was that this moment had come. Against all odds, denying the prognostication of the medical world, I had survived. Yes, I was injured and I was hurting, but I was alive.

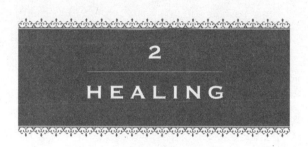

2

HEALING

THE MIRACULOUS BODY

While it is not the purpose of this exploration to embark on an anatomical analysis of the human body, nor to examine the nature of injury or illness, we must pause in reverence and pay homage to one monumental truth: The human body heals. Our body incorporates an astonishing ability to heal itself. Science can explain most, if not all, of how it happens, but we are not likely to ever know why. Religions, spiritual paths, and philosophies offer theories, but when it comes right down to it, the human body, while vulnerable, is simply miraculous.

The dictionary tells us that a miracle is a phenomenon that is not explicable by scientific or natural laws and is therefore often credited to a divine agency. That may or may not be. I, for one, am comfortable simply standing humbly in awe before what is so astonishing. The instant my body was so badly injured, it began to heal. If that is not miraculous, I do not know what is. It brings me to my knees.

Oh, what a beautiful and therapeutic tonic is gratitude. Gratefulness is not the only human experience, however, and like everything else, it is not immutable. Within a couple of days of leaving the hospital I entered into the most devastating, horribly despondent period of my life. I would not have believed that a basically happy, positive person could feel so miserable and hopeless. The depths of despair seemed limitless and the days endless.

The first morning at home, I stepped onto our scale and learned that I had lost twenty-five pounds. This was undoubtedly the result of two months without real food and exercise, added to the damage done by the severe burns. I was previously in good shape and I was now scrawny and physically weak. For those who might be tempted, let me state clearly that I do not recommend this type of "crash" diet (pun intended). Fortunately, I enjoy food, but gaining back this amount of weight in a healthful manner was not going to happen quickly. It took eight months to gain the first ten pounds and I still have a way to go.

I realized from that first day that my number one priority, for as long as it took, had to be my healing. More bluntly stated, I had to put me first. It felt like a strange and egocentric view and, I would like to believe, not my usual way of thinking, but the reality was stark and clear. If I did not recover, my life would be miserable and I would be of little use to anyone.

Susanna had considerable pain emanating from her broken vertebrae. She should have taken the same approach to her recovery as I did to mine, but my inability to attend to my basic daily needs meant that for the time being, she would be balancing my needs with her own. She was mobile, and other than no lifting or bending, she was able to lead a fairly normal life, albeit hampered by a heavy, restrictive, neck-to-waist brace, which she was to wear nonstop during waking hours.

Of the two of us, I had been the more seriously injured physically, and recovery was going to be challenging on every level—physical, mental, and emotional. I knew this, but I had no idea how formidable the actual journey was going to be. That challenge, the most daunting either of us had ever faced, would weigh heavily on both of us. Throughout the day I would want to lie down, not so much due to fatigue, although that certainly was part of it, but because of what is known as the "freeze mechanism." There are times when our options are fight, flight, or freeze. There was nothing and no one for me to fight, except myself. There was no place for me to flee and escape. The only remaining option was to freeze, which I did in the form of going to bed often and, I hoped, falling asleep. I did this for about two months, and then I stopped. I did not make a conscious decision to stop. I was just ready to move on.

I did not know at that time how close I had come to death. I was only to learn about that later. So, to be truthful, I was not constantly filled with gratitude. While I would be able in an occasional moment to feel the simple pleasures of life, mostly my days were filled with pain, dread, fear, anxiety, and the constant wish to have my life back. I felt as if I had no life. I thought it and said it so often: "I want my life back." It seemed as if there was nothing I could do for myself, and anything I attempted to do resulted in more pain and suffering. My hands were useless. I could not hold a fork or a toothbrush; I could not wash myself, dress myself, or wipe myself. I felt hopeless and life seemed pointless.

We can guarantee ourselves suffering when we cling to a desire for things to be different than they are. We can practically define suffering by saying that it is clinging to that desire. Things are *not* different than they are. They *are* as they are. Wanting things to change is not the same as putting out the effort and determination to bring about change.

I knew from my years of introspective practice that what I was experiencing were thoughts and feelings, and those thoughts and feelings were powerful, sometimes overwhelmingly so. So many mornings I woke up with the belief/hope that it had all been a dream and I was now back in my real life. Then I would stand up on my unsteady legs or try to use my painful hands and realize that this was no dream, a nightmare perhaps, but not a dream. This was now my life.

One day, in a moment of deep despair, Susanna, who was

going through the same kind of experience as I, said, "Now I can see that there are things worse than death. My beautiful life is gone. This life is horrible. It would have been better if we had died in the crash." I understood how she felt although I never quite reached the point of wishing I had died.

This was the most depressing, heartbreaking period of my life. There seemed to be no way out of the gloom. Perhaps that was the worst of it, the feeling that there was no way out. In the past, when there were difficult times, I was always able to find a solution. This was different. I had been seriously injured, and I was living with the consequences. I felt weak and broken. My vision, usually spacious and optimistic, had been narrowed and I could not see a broader picture. Susanna and I were living with physical pain and the suffering of witnessing each other's pain. She was hurting and devastated, and during this time I rarely found a way to help either of us. Often, at the end of a day, the best I could offer was, "Well, we made it through another day." It did not feel particularly positive, but in certain circumstances, survival is a triumph.

Like all phenomena, feelings that arise fade away. Thankfully, for the sake of our equanimity, we could acknowledge that we were extraordinarily fortunate. It seemed odd to have been so *un*fortunate, yet, at the same time, so fortunate. It was miraculous that I was alive and that Susanna could walk. A split second, or a centimeter one way or another, could have yielded a disastrous result. Doctors Tan and Yurt told us that the possibility of recovery, though far off in the distance, was real, and that *did* make a monumental difference.

SINCE THE accident I have focused primarily, but not exclusively, on my recovery. One special exception was the morning of

April 14, 2013, when I returned to teach at the Community Meditation Center, the spiritual home I had founded in 2008. At the suggestion of several CMC board members, I entered the building through a side door so that people would not "be all over me." When I was introduced, I walked smoothly and briskly to the front of the room, leaped (with a prayer) up onto the platform, and was greeted by the huge crowd with a standing, cheering, and tearful ovation. The more they cheered, the more I teared. It was an indescribable moment.

We admire survivors. We need survivors and those who have overcome the odds. The greater the odds they have overcome, the more we want to see them, to touch them, to hear their stories. We need to know it can be done. That is what I was that day and ever since. I had done it. I had survived.

DR. YURT'S team began speaking with me about my need for something called "Jobst garments." They anticipated that the garments could be of considerable benefit to me but acknowledged that there were some drawbacks. I began allowing the drawbacks to create a fair amount of anxiety within me. Jobst, it seems, is simply a trademark for a type of garment, or wrap, used to control hypertrophic scar formation (which applied to me) or lymphedema (which did not).[1] I had a considerable amount of scarring due to burns and the grafting and surgeries that followed. When issued by a hospital, these garments are measured meticulously for each individual patient. They are supposed to dramatically decrease the time it takes for scar tis-

---

[1] Hypertrophic scar formation deposits excessive amounts of collagen that result in a raised scar—in laymen's language, simply "scar." Lymphedema is a condition of localized fluid retention and tissue swelling caused by a compromised lymphatic system.

sue to be diminished. The down side, which brought about my anxiety, was about the reputed discomfort of these garments. To be effective, they had to fit very tightly and are supposed to be worn twenty-three hours a day. We were having these conversations in April 2013, with New York City's hot and humid summer months rapidly approaching. The thought of what amounted to a pair of long johns under my pants, plus skintight gloves, was less than appealing.

Nevertheless, I had myself measured for the garments, and they arrived three weeks later. To say that the pants were tight would be like saying that the Grand Canyon is a slit in the ground. I had another appointment scheduled for right after I was to try on the pants, so I had an eye on the clock. Therefore, I can report accurately, that with Susanna's assistance, Linda, a woman who helps people try on these garments every day, needed forty minutes to get one leg up to my knee. She explained that when brand-new, the pants are quite snug. (She is apparently a practitioner of understatement.) Things speeded up at this point, and within an hour the pants were on.

I then innocently asked, "What happens when I have to pee?" (It is always a difficult decision in a medical setting whether to say "urinate" or "pee." Linda seemed like a casual sort so I went with "pee.") Linda pointed out that there was an opening in front similar to that in men's underwear. I simply had to pull the opening open. When I reminded her of how weak and sensitive my hands were, and how tight the new garb was, she agreed that the whole concept of this garment needed to be reassessed.

The ever clever Susanna had the perfect solution: make two separate leggings that would go from the ankle to the top of the thigh. In addition, make two anklets, one for each ankle, since they had been particularly injured. I would be like a cowboy with chaps and spats. Three weeks later I received a call that the new garments were in and I could come try them on. My anxiety level rose, my hands perspired, and there was a knot in my stomach. If these material torture chambers fit this time, I would have to wear them.

I trembled my way over to the hospital and much to my surprise, not only did they slip on reasonably easily, but after thirty or so minutes I hardly noticed them. It turned out that I had little trouble wearing them twenty-three hours a day. It was yet another example of how easily one can create internal havoc and turmoil by projecting into the future and writing story lines that never happen. No wonder the idea of living in the present moment has been so honored for millennia. Fear and anxiety are feelings, and we can experience feelings only in the present. The fear we experience, however, is likely to be about something that has not yet happened, and perhaps never will.

As an example, here is a series of journal-type notes I wrote for myself during the summer of 2013:

August 12: I became extremely sad when I learned of the likelihood that part of my left pinky would have to be amputated. What we thought was necrotic tissue is more likely to be bone protruding through the front of the finger. That will have to be removed and perhaps most of the finger as well. Right now that is hitting me hard. My efforts are to focus on being in the present, but I am definitely struggling.

August 13: Throughout the day I consciously used my practice of being present, noticing as my mind was racing ahead with speculative thoughts regarding the protruding bone in my finger. Gradually, the gloom lifted. I have no way of knowing what the doctor will say tomorrow, so I might as well enjoy today. How easy that is to say, how difficult it is to practice.

August 14: I met with the hand surgeon today. He was conservative and essentially recommended watching and waiting. I had been told by one of my therapists that there was probably bone protruding from my left pinky. The doctor felt it was not bone. He could not identify exactly what it was, but whatever it was, even if bone, it would most likely dry up by itself and fall off. If it was painful or bothersome before that happened, he could remove it with a fairly simple procedure. (My experience has been that "simple procedures" are always done on someone else, not on one's self.)

August 25: Whatever was protruding from my left pinky fell off unassisted today.

I have spent most of my life worrying about things that have never happened.
——MARK TWAIN

I have heard the Dalai Lama suggest that if there is a problem and you can do something about it, there is no need to worry. If there is a problem and you cannot do anything about it, there is no point in worrying.

On the other hand (again, pun intended), there was the matter of compression gloves. Since my hands were heavily scarred, these gloves were recommended for the best possible healing. With my positive legging experience fresh in mind, I proceeded to my fitting without concern. (I also thought that the gloves, although flesh colored, might be noticed while out in public, and get me an occasional sympathetic glance. The leggings, not being visible, brought me only speedier and more thorough healing.) Truthfully, I never found the gloves to be completely comfortable, although they did get me the occasional concerned query: "Hey, dude, what's with the gloves? It's ninety-five degrees out." While I was never enamored of the gloves, they have been effective and the scars on my hands are slowly softening and flattening.

It is the nature of the body to heal. My occupational therapist, Eugenia, told me that in her view, all the people who were helping me, including her, were simply adjuncts to the process. I have worked with as many as five such adjunct-type people in a week. Every day, at home, I faithfully do the exercises prescribed by each. I fully believe that the body heals itself, but I also believe it can use all the help it can get.

The Dream Team

At the end of one of my regular biweekly exams in June 2013, Dr. Yurt said to me, "Okay, I'd like to see you in three months." My jaw must have dropped because he quickly added, "It's good. You are graduating." I did not feel like I was graduating; I felt like I was being abandoned. It was a deeply troubling feeling until I realized that, in a certain sense, he was not my doctor, he was my surgeon, and a superb one at that. I felt better when he made it clear that he understood my feelings of abandonment and that he would always be available for any questions related to my surgeries, grafts, or anything else within his ken. I also realized that my everyday medical needs during this recovery period would best be directed to my primary physician, who I now felt was more than my doctor, but a true friend.

The skin on both my legs had been grafted from the ankles to the tops of the thighs, making a considerable length of flesh susceptible to some serious itching. On a couple of occasions I experienced itching of such intensity that I had insights into what it must be like to feel as if you are going crazy. I was probably fortunate that my fingernails, which had melted away in the fire, had not as yet grown back, or I might have left myself with some significant scratch marks. There are times when our innate fight-or-flight mechanism simply cannot function, and all we can do is accept. In the case of this itching, Benadryl cream and well-focused deep breathing were of great value. It is still not known if my fingernails will actually grow back, but aside from a rather strange aesthetic appearance, I'm managing just fine. (What seems truly strange is that I no longer have fingerprints. They, too, apparently melted away. I do not seem to have a need for fingerprints, so no problem.)

Once home, our insurance allowed for a limited number of visits from a nurse who would do things like change my dressings, as well as a physical therapist and an occupational therapist. A home health aide was also provided for a limited number of hours per day for a few weeks. The nurse was fine, but ultimately, and pretty quickly, the time allocated by our insurer ran out and she faded from the picture. The occupational therapist was sweet and skillful, but the allotted home visits also ran out quickly. The physical therapist spent considerable time typing notes into her laptop but did always manage to get in a few minutes of therapy each session. We were told that the quality of the therapeutic sessions offered at the hospital was much better, so that was my next move.

Life being as life is, the skill, caring, and commitment of the therapists at the hospital also varied considerably. To be frank, what I found was that the younger, less experienced therapists were, well, young and inexperienced, and the older, more experienced ones often seemed bored. My injuries were, not surprisingly, of interest to me, unique, and with a quality all their own. How could anyone not be as fascinated by them as I was? While I can speak of this now with a smile, there were times when I felt unseen and unheard. In one particular session, I reported that my right shoulder was becoming tight, painful, and less mobile. The response from the therapist was, "Let's get on the leg press." We never did address my shoulder.

The irony of the combination of medical insurance and therapy is that, in order for the insurance company to continue to pay for your sessions, the therapist has to assure them that you are making progress. If you are making too much progress, however, the company will no longer pay for your sessions, this based on an assumption that you no longer need the therapy. I am not making this up. I was dropped from physical therapy because "You have made so much progress." The fact that I was too unsteady on my feet to walk outdoors by myself and my hands were too weak to turn on my electric toothbrush was apparently irrelevant.

I was learning that it was my responsibility to put together the right team for me. It did take some time and effort, and an occasional self-reminder that I did not want to hurt anyone's feelings, but I ultimately put together a supreme Dream Team. It was a group of skilled practitioners that quickly became invaluable to my healing.

Susanna, my wife and advocate, was the captain of the team, although I always kept in mind that she was injured also and was herself dealing with pain and serious trauma. As we counsel each other, I can see that our "former selves" are being burnished, not tarnished, by an unwanted but extraordinary twist in our lives.

THE SPECIFIC details of each situation will determine what skills are needed on the recovery team. We can use my situation as a guide. I had suffered severe burns and needed a surgeon/burn care specialist. I was incredibly fortunate, not just once, but twice. In Singapore, I was treated by Dr. Tan Bien Keem, a man whose remarkable medical skills and unbounded compassion have previously been discussed. I cannot claim to have made the decision to choose BK. I was unconscious when I was brought to him. Perhaps even in the darkest moments there can shine a light of such intensity that, conscious or not, good things will happen.

BK was the first physician who did not tell Susanna that I was going to die. He was instead the first to tell us that I could regain full function. Today, ninety-five hundred miles are not enough to keep us from staying in touch. More than a year after BK operated on me, he came to the United States for work and study. We met for a fabulous reunion over lunch and I asked him how he knew I would survive when every other doctor felt I could not. He said that when he cut into my body he could feel an energy—a life force—that was too powerful to die at that time. I remain in awe of his insight.

When I was flown by medevac to New York, I again landed in the hands of good fortune—more specifically, in the hands of an extraordinary surgeon. In my drugged state, I was placed in the care Dr. Roger W. Yurt, who is Chief of Burns, Critical Care, and Trauma at the New York–Presbyterian/Weill Cornell Medical Center. Every hospital and medical facility will claim "all of our doctors are excellent," but it quickly became clear to me that Dr. Yurt was "The Man." Although they might not own up to it now, when I quietly asked a couple of staff people who they would want as their doctor if the need arose, they quietly whispered, "Roger Yurt." If there is a particular doctor you want, do not hesitate to ask for him/her. You may not get your first choice, but there is no harm in trying.

My first choice as my occupational therapist was Eugenia. She is experienced, kindhearted, and willing to push me when it is for my own good. She bends, squeezes, pushes, pulls, massages, and cajoles my hands against their injured resistance. I can always see in her face that it is not pleasant for her to cause me pain, but her actions flow from a compassionate heart.

Aside from the actual burn injuries I sustained in the accident, my body had grown weak from two months of hospitalization. Physical therapy was called for. As I mentioned previously, my experience with the hospital's physical therapists was not satisfying. At the heart of the matter, it appeared to be that the system was more at fault than the individuals. As an example, if a therapist's session ended at three p.m. and her next one was scheduled to start at three p.m., obviously one had to end early or the other begin late. That might sound like a minor point, but with the sessions being only thirty minutes in length, three minutes lost amounted to 10 percent of the session. In some instances, therapists can be working with two or three patients at the same time. In that circumstance, attention to your individual needs is slim. I knew I could do better.

It did not take long for us to hear about Ginny, who has been a physical therapist for more than twenty years. What I really appreciate about her is that she pays careful attention, not just to how my body is functioning but to how I am experiencing that function. She listens to, and respects, my views. It is also pleasant to be around someone whose warm, infectious laughter is ubiquitous, not to mention that her fifty-five-minute sessions begin on time.

In the earlier part of this life, I enjoyed favorable results working with a psychotherapist, which was fortunate since I had a difficult childhood. My mother died when I was a teenager and my father suffered from a serious bipolar illness that made him abusive and often violent. Several times I accompanied the police as they escorted my dad to a psychiatric hospital. The last time he went awry, his neighbor called me and suggested that I come quickly. After driving speedily through the streets of Manhattan into the far reaches of Brooklyn, I arrived at his modest attached house. The shocking scene I came upon was taking place in the backyard. I moved quickly and was just able to pull Dad off a young woman he had pinned to the ground, while wielding an axe over her head. He was arrested and, nine days later, died in a forensic ward.

I am grateful for the work I did in therapy and that I now do in meditation. I believe these practices opened the door to the joyful and fulfilling experience that is my life. That does not mean every moment is a bubbly delight. That would be unrealistic. One thing it does mean, however, is that I am usually open to any type of mind/body exploration that can lead to greater insight and wisdom.

Until March 2013, I had never heard of Somatic Experiencing. Then, as if by coincidence (for those who believe in coincidences), several people whose opinions I trust suggested that I look into this relatively new form of psychotherapy, because it specifically addresses the issues brought about by trauma.[2] In view of the fact that this work has now played an invaluable role in my healing process, I would like for others who are dealing with trauma to know about it. Briefly, in layman's terms, Somatic Experiencing (SE) is a body-awareness approach to trauma, based on the understanding that human beings have an innate ability to overcome the effects of trauma.

The SE theory suggests that the symptoms of trauma are a result of a disruption of the autonomic nervous system.[3] It further posits that trauma has to do with the ways in which the mind/body system is overwhelmed when there is "too much, too soon" to be able to process. Emotions, behaviors, thoughts, images, and sensations all may accompany a given trauma and, with SE, the therapist emphasizes (but does not limit the work to) a focus on the nervous system and the unresolved, incomplete fight/flight/freeze responses as the seat of where trauma lives.

In SE, the body is the reference point and it is where one works to integrate whatever has shifted in the direction of healing. For example, if a person has an emotional shift, say from terror to greater ease, the person is invited to observe that shift

---

[2] Trauma is a natural response to a frightful event, such as an accident, rape, serious illness, loss of a loved one, or natural disaster. Immediately after the event, shock and dissociation are typical. Long-term reactions can include unpredictable emotions, flashbacks, strained relationships, and physical symptoms of many kinds, including headaches or nausea. While these responses to trauma are normal, some people have difficulty moving on with their lives.

[3] The autonomic nervous system functions primarily below the level of consciousness, controlling, among other things, digestion, respiratory rate, perspiration, salivation, and sexual arousal.

in the body, noticing whatever sensations convey the change in the physical state from terror to ease.[4]

Nancy is an extraordinarily gifted and experienced psychotherapist who has practiced Somatic Experiencing for some fourteen years. As she guides me through the challenging work of releasing trauma, she often reminds me, ". . . and you survived." The more deeply we dig, the more she reminds me, "You are here now. You survived."

Sometimes she suggests that I do some practice that seems odd to me. I give her a quizzical look and she smiles and says, "Okay, I know I'm a *whack job*." I told her about a TV commercial in which a rather sloppily dressed man is doing a wildly frenetic, highly ritualized dance in front of a television set. From the TV we hear a football game in progress. Then the home team scores a touchdown and the man watching the TV jumps for joy and celebrates. The following words appear on the TV screen: "It's only weird if it doesn't work."

When Nancy suggested that each day I take a few minutes to thank my hands for the hard work that they are doing in order to heal, it did seem rather strange to me. Then again, a touchdown is a touchdown and my hands are healing. I have made it a policy not to argue with what tastes scrumptious, no matter what ingredients are in the recipe.

THE WORK

The work involved in healing can be challenging. Depending on the extent of the trauma, illness, or injury, it can, in fact, be incredibly grueling. For our purposes, the work of healing, or

---

[4] Gratitude to Nancy Napier for this contribution.

recovery, refers to our efforts to return to normalcy and good health following a traumatic event, illness, or accident. It is intended to lead to either our previous way of living, or perhaps an even better and healthier life. To heal or recover is not the same as to be cured. An illness may end, but we may not feel fully recovered, or we may be completely recovered physically from an accident, but not as yet be free of the trauma it caused. We may be glad to be out of a particular relationship but still be dealing with the emotional turmoil brought on by the breakup. We may come to a point of acceptance with the fact that we have had a leg amputated but still be struggling with how to get around pain free. It is important to remember that there may not be a cure, but we can heal. There is a significant and far-reaching distinction.

A doctor's examination might find nothing wrong, but a recent loss may have left us with headaches, insomnia, depression, fatigue, and a lack of appetite. There is nothing that can be cured, but over time healing can come about through patience, self-compassion, and acceptance.

We are complex beings, and as such, there may not always be simple solutions to certain issues. Healing and recovery take place across the entire spectrum of human experience—physical, mental, and emotional. That is why, to use my case as an example, there had to be a fairly wide-ranging team of practitioner/therapists. Dealing with the loss of a loved one, the loss of a job, or an abusive relationship does not require an occupational therapist, but a psychotherapist could be invaluable. There is no way to get around one obvious fact. No matter who else is on the team, you are the one who will be doing the work. You are the center of your health care team. You are the Commander in Chief. Everyone else is an adjunct, valued and appreciated, but still an adjunct. Do not fret. There is more help available than you might imagine, good, competent, skillful, caring help. You are not alone.

AS STATED, one of the miracles of the human body is its ability to heal. It looks to find the most efficient route to return itself to its greatest functional state. Our role is to support that healing process in the wisest and most beneficial way. We begin by encouraging within ourselves clarity of mind and a positive attitude. This is most obvious as we address emotional issues, but is just as true when we are looking to heal from a physical illness or injury. Finding any and all ways to reduce stress is usually a good place to start the healing process.

Negative thinking is, by its very nature, a stressor, so finding any positive aspects of a current situation is likely to be beneficial. Finding greater clarity, reducing stress, and creating a positive view is more likely to be accomplished with the guidance of a qualified psychotherapist. It is important to realize that the therapist is a guide. It is your ship and you must steer it. To sit in the therapist's office week after week and not practice what you are learning is like studying a prescription given to you by a doctor but never taking the medicine. We complain, "I have been going to that therapist for a year but nothing has changed. She hasn't helped me." *You* must do the work. No teaching, no philosophy, no religion, no book, can do more than offer someone else's experience. The development of wisdom is the responsibility of each individual. If you believe that it is God who does the healing, that is fine, but the Divine will never turn down your well-considered assistance.

I BEGAN studying Tai Chi Chuan and that has been wonderful for my balance. I also find that the concentration required to perform the Tai Chi forms is rewarding on several levels, and I enjoy the work. Coming out of a traumatic event, we can easily forget that life can still be enjoyable. A number of years ago I was complaining to my dharma teacher about various things that were not going the way I wanted. When I finished my grumbling, she asked, "Are you at least enjoying all this misery?" It seemed an odd question at the time, but now I get it.

I have also found that getting back, as much as I could, to my professional life has been extremely healing. There may be nothing as therapeutic as a sense of normalcy, a feeling, even if it is only a feeling, that things are all right. I get great pleasure from teaching and writing. About six weeks after I came out of the hospital, one of my CMC students asked me if I would be willing to teach a small class of experienced meditators. I had some misgivings because I had no idea what my strength and concentration would be like. I agreed to try as long as the group was kept small and that they understood my circumstances. It turned out to be a wonderful idea. I was energized by their challenging questions and by the enthusiasm we shared.

I was learning that it is possible to deal with physical pain and the inconveniences caused by infirmities, while at the same time be productive and enjoy oneself.

RECEIVING

From the beginning we received many calls, cards, notes, e-mails, and texts with good wishes, prayers, and offers to help. Susanna would read them to me each day in the hospital and they provided a tremendous and often deeply moving lift. Sometimes the writer mentioned how much we meant to them, and at times, Susanna and I felt as if we were attending our own memorial service. We saw, yet again, how much a kind word can mean. I have also been reminded of how important friendships are in my life, and to have a friend I must be a friend. If I am too busy for a friend, then I am too busy.

I, like many others, am much more comfortable giving than receiving. With Susanna and me both being injured, we had to learn the graceful art of receiving. Most often the gift offered was food, one of the most basic and essential. Friends and neighbors would shop for us, sometimes without even asking what we needed. So many of them had been guests in our home and just seemed to know our tastes. Other times people cooked extra when preparing their meals and shared them with us. One Jewish family prepared beautiful, complete Sabbath meals and brought them to us on Friday evenings, ready to enjoy. Our paths might have been different, but the meals were fabulous. Other times, in fact at any time, full grocery bags would appear, hanging on the handle of our front door.

Two friends, with whom I have shared many joys and sorrows through the years, sent a techie to install and teach me how to use the dictation software they bought for me. The owner and all the employees of our favorite art gallery in Santa Fe went out shopping and each bought something special they thought we would enjoy. It all came in a large box, but it was the letter that they wrote, filled with such love, that moved us so deeply.

I do not consider myself a collector of watches, but I do have a few. I like watches that are subtle and graceful, and I particularly like those that keep truly accurate time. A friend was visiting and I happened to admire his watch. I asked if it kept accurate time and he commented that it kept *particularly* accurate time. Two days later a package arrived. He had bought me one of those watches.

A friend who was a regular at the CMC had moved from New York because, with her limited income, she found it so expensive. She sent us a letter saying how much she wished she was with us and could enfold us in her arms. Since she could not do that, she sent quite a large check instead. It was not easy figuring out how to return the check in the most honorable way, so I did what I often do in difficult situations. I asked Susanna to handle it, which she did with the utmost grace.

In the past I had enjoyed the pleasures of giving. Now, as a recipient (and in spite of our decision not to keep the above-mentioned check), I was clearly seeing joy in the faces of others as they became the givers. Seeing their delight helped me become more comfortable when receiving. There is also research suggesting that allowing in this type of love helps promote healing. I looked for any feelings of shame, unworthiness, or self-condemnation that might arise within me. It took a while, but I became comfortable with simply saying "Thank you" or "This means a lot" or "I really appreciate this." When I said these things, I meant them, and I accepted and appreciated that the giver/receiver relationship was contributing to my recovery. Ultimately, I believe that the giver and the receiver are as one. In reality there is no duality.

It was sobering and humbling to realize that some of our friends were doing things for me that I might not have done for others. The hospital to which I went for therapy was on the other side of the city from where I live. Public transportation, while possible, would have been long and quite inconvenient, especially for one who had just finished a taxing therapy session.

Susanna sent out a weekly e-mail to our friends who owned cars asking if, that week, anyone could pick me up. For our friends, that would typically mean going to their garage (which was never part of their home building), getting their car, and driving through New York City traffic. Often my sessions ran late, and since security would not allow anyone to park in front of the hospital, my friends would have to circle around, again through NYC traffic, until I appeared. Then they would drive me home (through NYC traffic). Next they would drive their car back to the garage (through NYC traffic) and return to their home by public transportation (through NYC traffic) or on foot (through NYC cell phone–wielding pedestrians). That round trip had to take at least an hour to an hour and a half. Yet every week one of them was there to pick me up. Is it any wonder that every one of those rides was to me a sacred journey?

TRANSITIONS

Desire change. Be enthusiastic for that flame
in which a thing escapes your grasp
while it makes a glorious display of transformation.[5]
—RAINER MARIA RILKE

In the truest sense, on a cellular level, we are always in transition. Everything is in a constant state of change. Nothing is fixed, permanent, or immutable. This ongoing state of rising and falling was seen some twenty-five hundred years ago by the Buddha when he taught that a characteristic of all phenomena is that of impermanence. At approximately the same time, the

---

[5] *Sonnets to Orpheus*, II, 12 (stanza 1), translated by Br. David Steindl-Rast.

Greek philosopher Heraclitus (ca. 535 BCE–475 BCE) noted, "No man ever steps in the same river twice, for it is not the same river and he is not the same man." Contemporary research concurs that all things are constantly in a state of change.

Generally speaking, we do not tend to be particularly comfortable with change, even when the change is moving us toward that which we view as preferable to our current state. Discomfort, whether perceived as gross or subtle, is referred to in the ancient language of Sanskrit as *dukkha* (suffering, unhappiness, dissatisfaction, sadness, unrest, grief, and so forth). The entire Buddhist philosophy is based on acknowledging the existence of dukkha, identifying its cause, and the truth that we can bring about its cessation, thus achieving awakening, freedom, and abiding happiness. In the practice of meditation we can quietly observe the nature of change as we note the arising and dying away of phenomena. In this practice we see our thoughts, feelings, and sensations appear as if from nowhere, and then fade away, to where, we do not know. But that is always the pattern: what arises (birth), fades away (death). It is true of you and me; we have been born and we will die. Oddly enough, a hundred years from now there will be no one on this earth who ever knew us.

This insight may at first be disconcerting, but truth can be invaluable as we look to free ourselves from the habitual patterns of clinging and grasping. After all, what are we trying to hold to so tightly? Whatever it is can never truly be ours. It either dies away first, or we die away first.

About six months after my accident, I noticed an interesting conflict going on within me. I had made considerable progress on all levels, and while there was obviously a long way to go in terms of complete healing, I was essentially doing with my life what I wanted to do. I was enjoying my family and friends, and I was involved in, and excited about, my teaching and writing. Yet, when someone asked me how I was feeling, I noticed some reluctance on my part to say, "I feel good" or "I'm doing well, thank you." I found that curious, since I never wanted to be seen or thought of as *Allan who was injured*, or *the man who was in a plane crash*. I want only to be seen and accepted for who I am, fallibilities, scars, and unskillfulness included.

At the same time, I felt a certain desire to make sure that the other person knew what I had been through and that the challenges I faced were by no means over. I offered a detailed account of the accident any number of times. This dichotomy became a matter for exploration in meditation, and while the investigation continues, I have decided to explore answering the "How are you feeling?" question with a cleaner, more direct response. Invariably, that reply has become a simple, "I feel good. Thank you." That answer is almost always true and is usually what the inquirer enjoys hearing. While that might not be a complete answer, on a given day, even if I do not feel particularly good, I am still able to say that overall I am doing better. Those with whom I feel particularly close might get a more detailed answer, but whether my reply is brief or detailed, I make sure that it is truthful. I now find that I am residing more regularly on the positive side of the transition.

With that, I would add that I am surprised at how long the pain has continued in my hands. I was told early on that the physical healing process would take up to two years, yet I am still amazed when I have days of ongoing pain, or intermittent sharp, stabbing pains. By the end of one of those days I might feel weary, yet I am still okay. I am buoyed by the fact that I have made it through the day and tomorrow might be easier.

With enough tomorrows, the healing process will have run its course.

It seems to me that without making that kind of transition, one can easily be trapped in a state of incomplete healing. Even if the pain has ended and health has been restored, the need to relate often to the traumatic event, or illness, is likely to be detrimental. It would be easy to build an identity, or an image, as a victim. My preference is to think, speak, and act as the healthy person I am, even as my scars are healing.

I am not at all enamored of the phrase "get over it." Unless one has the professional training and is asked to evaluate when it might be wise for someone to move on, it is probably best that individuals be allowed to determine their own progress. The suggestion here is more about being aware, noticing what is going on in the mind and body, and becoming more mindful of where the mind is leading you. Encourage the mind to direct your recovery. Thoughts of lovingkindness and compassion directed toward your self can be of great benefit. Your recovery and good fortune do not take from anyone else. In fact, a healthy you makes for a more healthy world.

Shambhala Sun, a beautifully produced, Buddhist-oriented magazine, did an interview with me in February 2014. The photographer was talented and I enjoyed working with her. When I saw the photos it was evident that she was truly a high-end professional. Nevertheless, my heart sank. I had become accustomed to how I looked during this transitional period and the daily glance in the mirror yielded no surprises. Staring at those photos, however, allowed me to see where I actually was at this point. There were still the remains of scars on my head. There was still a piece of one ear missing. There was still quite a contrast in color where grafting had been done. There was definitely a little jolt of reality, but happily it did not last long. We have little if any objectivity when it comes to our own appearance, and in my case, I realized that I was fortunate to have any appearance at all.

We are all in transition and we are all in some state of healing. Mirrors and photos reveal certain truths, and with maturity we learn how to see what is true within the truth.

Pain

Unfortunately, transitions do not necessarily move in a logical or linear fashion. In the process of healing, we are most likely making physical progress every day, but it may not necessarily feel that way. In any given moment it may feel as if we are not moving forward and will never do so again. We may feel emotionally bereft, as if recovery is just an illusion, like a lake in the desert, a mirage that calls to us but can never assuage our thirst. I have had many such days. The pain in my hands sometimes presents itself as sharp and stabbing, and at other times it resides all day as low-level soreness and twinges. I understand that it is part of the healing—specifically, in my case, the regeneration of nerves. Nevertheless, physical pain is compelling. It can grab us by the throat and tarnish the luster of the day. (A nice way of saying, *it can hurt like hell*.)

Of all the questions people ask when I teach, the ones that come up most often relate to dealing with physical pain. I wish I had easy answers, but the complex nature of the human psycho/physical organism, combined with the intricacies that the sensations of physical pain comprise, make a simple, easeful solution unrealistic. Also, quite frankly, I never felt I had the necessary personal experience to address the subject of serious, chronic pain with a depth of expertise. I have had scratches and cuts, sprains and strains, a root canal, and an arthroscopic surgery or two (too much tennis), the same as everyone else. I even had a kidney stone removed. But I had never experienced a serious illness or injury within my own body for a sustained period of time until that plane plunged from the sky.

Now that has changed. It is not a change I sought or desired. Nevertheless, pain, discomfort, and distress have become my close companions. Since Christmas Day 2012, they have been with me every day, and I have come to know them intimately. Sometimes they stay for the entire day, and other times they drop in for quick, intense visits. Many are the days we wake up together, shower and shave together, eat meals, do chores, work and play, and go to bed together. Sometimes, as the clock ticks and the sky darkens, we spend sleepless hours together in the middle of the night, as I engage with pain's relentless besiegement.

I have gained new insights into "The Middle Way," the path that allows us to accept, and at the same time aggressively battle, these unwelcome visitors. It is a tough road, at times bloody and discouraging. The pain still hurts, that is the nature of pain; but we can change our relationship to the painful sensations, and that can make an enormous difference.

Start by letting go of the idea that pain is an enemy. It is not, and it is best not to create unnecessary adversarial relationships. We experience all phenomena as either pleasant or unpleasant. Pain is a label for a series of sensations that we usually find unpleasant. Because of their unpleasant nature, our tendency is to want to stop the sensations, to push them away, and we want to do so as quickly as possible. We are inundated with advertisements for products that, we are told, will obliterate our pain faster and more effectively than any other. When we cannot do that, we often become annoyed and resentful. If the situation continues long enough, we can become bitter.

Even though the painful sensations are unpleasant, we can learn to view the experience with acceptance and self-compassion. In my case, as an example, pain in my hands can serve as a reminder that I still have my hands and all of my fingers, which I will never again take for granted. They were severely burned in the accident, and two fingers came close to being amputated. None of my fingers function normally as yet, but they are progressing, and each day I thank my fingers and hands for working so hard to heal. I began this practice at the suggestion of my trauma (Somatic Experiencing) therapist. I will admit that at first it felt a bit hokey to speak to my hands, but the more I gave myself over to it, the more effective I found it to be. It took me a while to speak to my hands gratefully and with sincerity. I knew that just mouthing words would be meaningless.

I have a pretty good skeptical streak within me, but I do not argue with success. It is quite clear that acceptance, gratitude, and compassion soften me, while anger, bitterness, and aversion tighten me. If nothing else, I feel a certain ease course through my body when I practice gratitude. It feels very different from the tightness of aversion. (Since I want to retain some semblance of sanity I speak to my hands only when no one else is around. And to be clear, my hands do not answer me. It is said that if a man speaks to God, he is holy. If God speaks to him, he is psychotic.)

Some things heal only in their own time. My right index finger was seriously injured and I was left with a dead fingernail surrounded by necrotic tissue. It made the finger not very useful, although I was extremely grateful to still have it. Exactly fifty-four weeks after the accident, the nail and the dead tissue fell to the floor in a bloody lump. It was a bit sore but now I am gaining more and more use of the finger, and consequently the hand. It was a matter of time and the miraculous body doing its thing.

IT IS perfectly natural to want to push away or cover over unpleasant sensations, but that does not mean it is our best, or only, option. We can change our relationship to pain by learning about its true nature, not by running from it or constantly medicating ourselves. This is a radically different concept for most people because we are so conditioned to grasp immediately for anything that will stop the unpleasantness. We also live in a society whose economic health is grounded in our desire to pursue pleasure. To be clear, there are times when the wisest and most compassionate action is the use of appropriate medication, but we must also acknowledge that as a society we are conditioned to overmedicate.

It takes practice to develop the skills that allow us to gain insight into the true nature of things, and that is definitely the case when it comes to learning about the true nature of physical pain. We begin that practice by inviting the entire body to become as calm as possible. Then we bring a gentle but precisely focused awareness to the area of the pain. We call this "single-pointed focus." This step may well feel counterintuitive if previously our approach has been to cover up pain as quickly as possible. Now we are looking directly at the sensations that we label "pain." We see that "pain" is simply a name that we have agreed to use to represent unpleasant sensations. Now, what can we learn about those sensations? Are they sharp or are they dull? Do they stay in one place, or are they moving around? Are they hot, or are they cold? Can you feel the vibrations? (They *are* vibrating.) What is their color? What is their shape? What other characteristics can you notice? Take your time; look carefully with a "beginner's mind" at the minute details.

You are not trying with this practice to eliminate pain but to change the way you experience it. Pain is vibration. Under certain conditions, the vibrations can be unpleasant, and when persistent, they can seem intolerable. Remember that your mind is your most powerful ally, and you can be persistent also. You can be calm and determined. You are an intelligent being and you know that in each moment everything is changing. Watch those changes in the sensations. Perhaps you will even see them ease, perhaps not. You will see that you can handle the situation. You will win. To be sure, there are times when medication is the wisest choice, but it does not always have to be our first choice.

When we are going through difficult times, especially if physical pain is involved, it can be easy to forget to be grateful for what is working well. Because pain can be so compelling, it can quickly plunge us into depths where all seems bleak. It is important that we resist that pull and develop skills that help us combat the powerful force of physical pain. The graciousness of gratitude is a magnificent ally, as well as being a sincere expression of an enlightened being.

Remember that no one is more worthy of your love and tenderness than you are yourself. I think it is unfortunate that so many of us were raised to believe that we are unworthy. That simply is not true and is an unskillful way to think. Unskillful thinking leads us toward suffering and distress, while skillful thinking leads us toward inner peace, happiness, and awakening. This may be the time to reexamine and accept your own goodness, potential, and worthiness. It is powerful medicine and can heal like no other.

This is not theory, philosophy, or religious dogma. It is my own hard-earned personal experience. I have been there with you. One-third of my body was seriously burned, some of it all the way to the bone. I know pain. I have been in the fire and I have come through the flames. Doctors said I would not live. They meant well, but they were wrong. I am healing. You can too.

DETERMINATION

As we navigate the path of healing and recovery it becomes evident that there are two qualities that we will need in abundance if we are to alleviate our pain and suffering. These two virtuous attributes are patience and determination. Often it will require determination to remain patient and, likewise, it may require patience to remain determined. As our model, let us look back almost twenty-five hundred years ago where, in northern India, a young man named Siddhartha Gautama was enjoying a life of ease and luxury. While he appeared to have it all—wealth, comfort, prestige—deep within he began to sense that he was missing some essential part of what life was about. He was so consumed by this spiritual void that he made the difficult decision to leave his home and loved ones in search of a greater truth.

He sought out and studied with the most renowned teachers. He practiced extreme austerities, which at that time in India many believed to be the "holy way," the way to enlightenment. (Even today, some still follow the path of severe deprivation.) His teachers were impressed with his intelligence and dedication, but after six years of study and practice he still felt he had not reached his goal, that of complete awakening.

His long journey on foot continued, and when he came to

the small town of Gaya, he sat down beneath an old sacred fig tree (*Ficus religiosa*).[6] Although he was likely exhausted, he was no less determined than the day he started out. He sensed that he was close to his goal and resolved not to get up from under that tree until he was a fully awakened being. The story goes on to tell how, throughout the long night, Mara arose within Siddhartha again and again. Mara is seen as the destroyer of virtuous pursuits, a demon that today might be known as "egoism." It breeds doubt, fear, distress, greed, and ignorance, to name but a few of its unpleasant traits. Mara can be a powerful foe and present a major challenge to our resolve and determination. This fiend exists within us all and encourages unskillful thinking (meaning that which leads to suffering), unkind words, and destructive actions.

At this point, Siddhartha had become wise to the ways of Mara. He recognized each assault and temptation for what it was, and each time it arose within him he simply said, "I know you, Mara." He combated the inner enemy by recognizing it for what it was. He did not get caught up in his emotional inner landscape but rather recognized his thoughts as thoughts, feelings as feelings, and sensations as sensations. He knew that he did not have to accept these phenomena as reality. We too can learn that we do not have to believe everything we think.

Siddhartha's resolve reaped great rewards, not only for himself but for all beings ever since. He overcame his doubts and fears and reached his goal of complete awakening. For the next forty-five years he taught what he had learned. His insights into the nature of suffering, its cause (which he saw as endless craving and clinging), and a pragmatic path that can bring peace to one's

---

[6] Gaya is approximately 218 miles from Lumbini, Siddhartha's birthplace.

heart and mind, remain a contribution to the world that is immeasurable.

Determination is the perseverance to stay the course, even when it feels as if we are drowning in doubt and misgiving. There may be times when we need the complete depth of our determination and tenacity. This level of courage is often accompanied by a sense of joy, because although the task is formidable, we sense that we are moving forward, toward wholeness. Determination strengthens determination.

Marci was twenty-five years old when she came to me to study meditation. A year before, her mother had died of breast cancer, and now she had been diagnosed with the same illness. She told me that although she was frightened, her fear was nowhere near as strong as her determination to win the battle. About six weeks later she said that, at first, all she wanted was to return to her normal life. Now, that was not good enough. If all she did were to return to where she was, she would have gained nothing from her illness. She wanted to live with greater insight and to be in the world as a better person. Her treatment and recovery went smoothly, and I believe her vision and determination were major factors.

What would you have to give up to be free from anger, turmoil, and negative feelings? The reality is that in this world, terrible things happen. Accidents, illnesses, tornados, fires, and earthquakes occur and can leave misery and suffering in their wake. When we are victimized, we can become angry—angry with a parent, an attacker, our body, or our God. Long after our physical pain subsides, our suffering continues. Yet at a certain point, we can make a transformative decision. Although victimized, we no longer have to think of ourselves as victims.

Even though it can manifest in various parts of the body, the only place fear can exist is in the mind. It is an important part of our practice to do battle with our fears. We may think sometimes that we are not making progress, but as long as we work diligently with skillful awareness and determination, we are advancing. Honor and courage are inherent within the struggle.

Determination can only be practiced in the present moment. Thinking ahead about how determined you will be tomorrow is not as effective as being determined in this very moment. When you want to quit because the pain and exhaustion are so intense, that is when you need to rouse determination. I know what that level of despair feels like. I have lived it and it is awful. Yet it has worked for me to dig in and not quit, and that is why I know in my heart it can work for you as well. Quitting on your self is likely to mean living out this life with bitterness. Quitting altogether opens a door that is best left closed. William Shakespeare was no fool and in his most famous soliloquy addresses the question of "Why live?" His sobering answer is that life, even at its worst, is still life. Death is unknown.

To be, or not to be, that is the question:
Whether 'tis nobler in the mind to suffer
The slings and arrows of outrageous fortune,
Or to take arms against a sea of troubles,
And by opposing end them? To die, to sleep,
No more; and by a sleep, to say we end
The heartache, and the thousand natural shocks
That flesh is heir to, 'tis a consummation
Devoutly to be wished. To die, to sleep;
To sleep, perchance to dream; Aye there's the rub,
For in that sleep of death, what dreams may come,

When we have shuffled off this mortal coil,
Must give us pause.[7]

Determination is a mental quality. Just as we can train the body, we can train the mind. It is your mind and you will see that you are equal to the challenge.

When you have come as close to dying as I have, you notice more readily when people complain about traffic, rainy days, slow elevators, long lines at the market, telephone solicitations, and others of life's annoyances. You realize that while the world might not be perfect, it is a good thing, a great and wondrous thing, as it is to be alive and weaving your imperfections with those of the rest of humanity.

PATIENCE

The best reply to unseemly behavior is patience and moderation.
—MOLIÈRE, *French dramatist,* 1622–73

It seems to be a matter of considerable curiosity among my friends and colleagues as to how patient I have been during this long and arduous period of recovery and healing. Some jokingly point out that I am the person who literally wrote the book on patience.[8] I am certain that the extensive time I spent studying the nature of patience and then writing about it has served me extremely well. While I have had to deal with many

---

[7] *Hamlet*: Act III, Scene 1, by William Shakespeare.

[8] Allan Lokos, *Patience: The Art of Peaceful Living* (New York: Tarcher/Penguin, 2012).

issues during this recovery, I believe that I have remained patient throughout. That would not have been the case a few short years ago.

For patience to develop you will need forbearance, tolerance, the ability to accept the truth, and most important of all, you will need to be cool. If that seems overwhelming, remember that your motivation is your desire for inner peace. As you progress, you develop faith that you can ultimately accept that which you cannot change.

For many, the most difficult person with whom to be patient is one's self. Patience with self is essential if we are to enjoy happiness and equanimity through life's constantly changing nature, with its unfair and disruptive conditions. We want to encourage acceptance, open-mindedness, compassion, and generosity of spirit within ourselves.

It is patience that protects us, and our loved ones, from the perils of our own anger, loss of compassion, and reactive behavior. Many of us are perfectly willing to say, "I have no patience for cell phones in elevators, drivers constantly honking their horns, right wing/left wing [you choose] political views." Yet ultimately we will be happier if we encourage within ourselves acceptance, open-mindedness, and compassion. Patience allows life to feel more spacious and easeful.

Terrible things happen in life and there is often no one to blame, but we blame anyway. We blame the boss, we blame the traffic, we blame inflation, we blame the doctor. When all else fails, we blame our God. We blame so much that we have become the most litigious society in history.

Those we find difficult, those for whom we feel aversion, whom we would prefer to avoid, are among our most important colleagues if we are to advance on this journey. It is with them that we transform theory and philosophy into virtuous action. It is with them that we learn patience.

When we are angry we are not happy, and we are more likely to suffer *dis*ease, *dis*comfort, and *dis*pleasure. To develop greater patience, we need to be aware of the presence of impatience and anger as they arise. To do that, we practice mindfulness. When we are aware of anger or impatience as they arise, we can see that they are feelings—feelings that exist within us. We do not have to justify feelings by trying to make them into reality. They are simply feelings.

WHEN WE are dealing with an illness, a loss, or recovering from an injury, the stress brought on by anxiety or physical pain may contribute to exacerbating impatience. That is perfectly understandable and we can offer our selves compassion. We can also view this as a time for deeper practice and the opportunity for greater insight.

When we speak or act while impatient, we dramatically increase the possibility that we will later regret our words and actions. We may very well even slow down that which we are trying to speed up. The process of healing will most likely advance more smoothly and efficiently as we practice greater patience. This personal development requires an understanding of the root causes of our stress, anxiety, and frustration, all of which can manifest as impatience. Then we must be willing to relinquish the type of thinking that leads to the loss of patience. It is not enough to say, "Of course I'm impatient. I'm lying here with severe pain. What do you expect?" Or, "Yes, I'm impatient. I feel like I'm going to vomit every five minutes. You would lose your patience too."

These are conditioned responses, no doubt legitimate,

generated by terrible circumstances. Nevertheless, greater patience can be developed even under the most trying of conditions. Then we will not respond with the type of emotional reaction that can cause more suffering for ourselves and others. To be sure, it would be much wiser to establish a depth of patience before a serious need arises. That means starting to work on patience now.

The vehicle for this kind of endeavor is called "mindfulness." We can think of mindfulness as a wholesome, moment-to-moment, nonjudgmental, nonclinging, engaged level of awareness. It is mindfulness that enables us to sense within ourselves the arising of feelings and emotions such as impatience and anger at their initial stirring and to calmly invite patience to come to the fore. We can do that with a practice as simple as saying to ourselves, "Patience." That is a simple practice, but remembering to do it is not necessarily easy. The word "practice" is both a noun and a verb. We must practice a practice for it to be effective.

In the research I conducted before writing *Patience: The Art of Peaceful Living*, I found that the number one reason people gave for "losing their patience" was a feeling of not being seen, or not being heard. When we are impaired, that sense of not being seen or heard can easily become heightened. We might experience so much impatience that we assume we are an impatient person. We say of ourselves, "I don't have a lot of patience," as if to suggest that we are hardwired a certain way and cannot change. We now know, not just theoretically or philosophically, but through exhaustive and thorough research, that everything and everyone is changing in every moment. No one is simply a patient or impatient person. That is too simplistic a view for such complex beings as we are.

Some of us refer to ourselves as "an angry person," ignoring that the basic nature of sentient beings is kind and compassionate. It is essential to understand that impatience and anger are feelings, real feelings, but they should not be viewed as reality. Like all other phenomena, feelings that arise fade away. They will always do that; it is their nature. We do not want to characterize ourselves based on a feeling. Teenage-type statements such as, "I would never . . ." or "I am the kind of person who . . ." would be more accurate if reframed as "to this point in my life, I have never . . ." or "I have usually favored . . ."

Patience is not a commodity or an item. You cannot run out of it. Patience is a feeling, and there is a significant difference between a feeling and a material object. The sense that we have "run out of patience" is simply an awareness of the arising of impatience. Again, remember that it is the nature of feelings to arise and then fade away. In the case of feelings like impatience and anger, it is often wise to help them fade away. We do not do that by denying their existence but by becoming aware of their deleterious effect on us.

Those who equate patience with weakness and anger with strength need to look again. Patience requires wisdom, courage, and compassion. It is a noble virtue, and essential if we are to know inner peace.

Perseverance, while of great value, is not true patience. It is more like the skills we learned as children that are intended to get us through challenging moments. They are the "take a deep breath and count to ten" or "remember, this too shall pass" practices that prevent us from causing or perpetuating stress with a conditioned response or knee-jerk reaction. They are simple tools, but they are valuable. They keep us from making reactive comments or acting out while annoyed, comments and actions that we would likely regret later on. A quick dose of perseverance may not feel particularly enlightened, but it can be invaluable while we do the work to develop deeper levels of true patience.

The more we cling to a desire for life to be different, the more likely we will experience impatience. Self-pity, despair, and blame will all be lurking in the shadows. Forbearance, on the other hand, includes a spirit of forgiveness. When the Buddha pointed out the truth of suffering, he was not saying that we should do nothing to alleviate it—quite the contrary. Patience is not passive. We are motivated by compassion for our own suffering and that of all beings.

Patience is born when we create a pause between a feeling that arises within us and our response to that feeling. Without a pause, we will most likely react in our conditioned manner. That is what conditioning is. With a pause, there is the possibility of a more positive response, and certainly we are less likely to cause harm with one of our ever-so-clever snarky comments. If we spend time with our experiences—the thoughts, feelings, and sensations that arise—we can gain insight. If wisdom can be defined as seeing things as they really are, we can say it develops as we see things with greater clarity.

When we truly see and accept that the experience of sentient beings includes aging, illness, and death, we can relax a bit with that reality; it is the way things are. You have done nothing wrong. You are not being punished. This acceptance does not mean that we do not make efforts to alleviate suffering. It means that with patience, we choose words and take actions that are well considered. Patience, contrary to popular misconception, is not characterized by passivity or indifference. It is alive, vital, and active. It is compassion for oneself and others.

Perseverance and endurance can help us avoid reacting with anger when we feel frightened, or when the inefficiencies of others cause unnecessary delays. With practice you will find that you can be mindful and take time to consider your responses. Even a momentary pause can help you see things more clearly and perhaps open up a different perspective, or an understanding of another person's situation. No wonder dharma teacher and psychotherapist Tara Brach refers to this moment as a "sacred pause."

It is likely that you will only be able to create such a pause if you decide that it is important to you. Without that firm decision and the dedication to back it up, the pull of habit, energy, and conditioning will continue to rule. For me, that decision is about a sincere desire to live life as the person I want to be. During my long and arduous period of healing, I am tested every day by pain and inconvenience. I don my mask and cape and do battle with my demons, armed only with my weapons of patience, compassion, and determination. I do not win every battle, but I am winning the war.

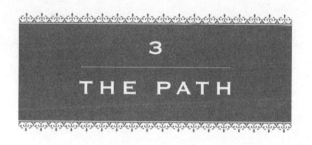

3

THE PATH

Whatever one reflects upon frequently becomes the inclination of the mind.

—THE BUDDHA, *Dvedhavitakka Sutta*

It was evident early on that I was recovering more quickly than anyone had anticipated. The healing road would be long and difficult, but rather than needing six months in the ICU as had been estimated, I was home in two months. I had trouble relearning how to walk, but once I caught on, I improved steadily. Even though my hands still have a long way to go before they are pain free and fully functional, I can cut food, get some use of the computer keyboard, dress myself, and sign my name.

As a longtime practitioner of Buddhist meditation, I am frequently asked how my practice has helped me during this trying time. I was also asked more than once if I felt that my practice played a role in my surviving the crash itself. The more I thought about these questions, the more I was reminded of just how deep, multifaceted, and profound meditative practices can be. Buddhism focuses primarily on one's state of mind, and our state of mind in a traumatic situation is of primary importance. When I was caught in the fire struggling to free myself, I knew my situation was dire and I was desperately frightened, but at the same time I believe my efforts were successful because I remained calm. Likewise, once I had jumped from the plane, those who helped me to safety also spoke of my composed demeanor.

How our mind perceives and guides us through the myriad challenges of healing is the single most important factor in determining how successful our efforts will be. Some aspects of the practices that we will now examine may seem more significant than others, but my experience has been that in a given moment what might otherwise seem inconsequential can, in another moment, be monumental.

MEDITATION

When I am asked what is the most significant practice that led me from the brink of death back to a joyful and thriving life, my first answer invariably is the practice of meditation. It is the foundation for all that works well in my life, and it is a major factor in my still having a life. It was certainly a most significant determinant in my being able to function quickly and calmly in a frightening situation.

For many years I have begun each day with meditation practice. I like to start my session by setting an intention. An intention, in this context, is simply a brief thought that helps us remember why we are meditating that day. I keep my intention concise, honest, and straightforward, not lofty and idealistic. It is not intended to help me correct all evils in the world. It might be as simple as "may I be kind throughout this day" or "may I be patient." As one who practices in the Buddhist tradition, I also take refuge mentally in "The Three Jewels": the Buddha (awakened one/the teacher), the Dharma (the teachings), and the Sangha (the community of noble beings who have walked this path before me. Today, "sangha" also denotes any group of people who meditate together or who gather to study the dharma).

Setting an intention each day may alleviate the repetition that can over time make practice drab. It also invites creativity and thoughtfulness. Meditation is a skill, and practicing it can be enjoyable in the same way as mastering any other meaningful skill.

Saying that meditation can be enjoyable does not mean that

it will always be easy. Every meditator knows it requires effort to sit through a session when unpleasant feelings are coming up. Uncomfortable physical sensations can also arise, adding to the experience. If we can view these challenges calmly and without self-criticism, the struggle eases and we gain insight. In this practice we face our issues and look honestly at any unskillfulness. We see that our thinking and our actions may not always be as wise as we previously thought.

Today, meditation and other mindfulness practices have become popular, and with popularity there is the possibility of commercialization and the diminishing of integrity. According to the National Institutes of Health, more than thirty million people claim to use meditation as some sort of treatment. It would be wonderful if meditation could cure all ills, repair broken bones, relieve constipation, and clear up acne. Any such claims should be examined with eyes fully open.

One thing we have learned in recent years is that there is no illness known to humankind that is not exacerbated by stress. The fact is that meditation, when practiced in the classical manner requiring that we stop other activities and focus the mind on the present, will in itself reduce stress. However, the practice is not about sitting and doing nothing. Focusing the mind is not as easy as it might sound. But research has shown that meditation may, in certain instances, be beneficial in dealing with anxiety, physical pain, and depression. Meditation is about actively training the mind so that we can live mindfully, become more aware of what is happening in the present, and alleviate suffering. Out of this is born wisdom and the first steps on the path of awakening.

Meditation, as taught by the Buddha some twenty-five hundred years ago, is not about stress reduction or curing maladies, other than the illness of delusion. Meditation was practiced for the purpose of gaining insight and wisdom so that the practitioner could see into the true nature of phenomena including the "self." Through this process we see how we create suffering for ourselves and those around us. Thus seeing, we realize that we can bring an end to such suffering. That rare but attainable state, the complete extinction of suffering, is called "Nirvana."

Innovative thinkers such as Dr. Jon Kabat-Zinn have been able to bring the ancient approach to meditation into the modern world in a way that remains authentic. His program, Mindfulness-Based Stress Reduction (MBSR), has been a blessing for tens of thousands of individuals. More than a decade earlier, in the 1970s, it was pioneers Joseph Goldstein, Jack Kornfield, and Sharon Salzberg who brought the ancient teachings to the West when they established the Insight Meditation Society in Barre, Massachusetts.

Even though the extinction of suffering remains a distant goal for most of us, every little step, every moment of insight, every flash of clarity, is filled with such fascination that it makes the journey wondrous. This path to happiness is not one in which we pursue pleasure. It is rather one in which we bring about the end of suffering through insight and wisdom, leaving us with a sense of inner peace and abiding happiness. In the process of recovering from trauma, any reduction in stress would be most welcome. I may have been in a serious accident that thrust me close to death and left me reeling with pain and despair, but I avoided worsening the situation by not creating additional suffering.

Happiness is a skill that can be learned. It requires time, effort, and patience, but we can adjust our thinking and perceptions and, in so doing, find the most positive view of all situations. That is not by any means to say that all events and situations are wonderful, but we are not helpless victims of our circumstances. Our entire quality of life can be impacted by minimal mental adjustments. We do not want to be held captive by our thoughts and emotions.

A powerful method for achieving this freedom is called "*Vipassana*," or insight meditation. The complex matrix of the human mind/body experience can be deeply appreciated during this practice. In the beginning, short practice sessions are fine. Five minutes a day can soon be extended to ten and then twenty. To practice, choose a quiet place and let others know you would like not to be disturbed. Turn off the television, radio, and telephones. If you are recovering from an injury, you may have to be creative as to your physical position when meditating. You have many options since the traditional positions are sitting, standing, walking, and lying down. (If lying down, be aware of the tendency to fall asleep. Sleeping is not meditating.) Let your hands rest comfortably on your lap, and once they are set, let them remain still throughout the session. Most meditators prefer to have their eyes closed, which eliminates visual distractions. (Even with eyes closed we see forms, colors, and movement.)

Start by sitting in a dignified, comfortable, and alert position, with back straight. Rest your awareness on an object of concentration. Traditionally, that "object" would be the sensations of the breath. It will be your anchor. (It may seem a bit odd to refer to a nonmaterial phenomenon as an object, but it is just traditional language—a convention.) Every time the mind wanders, return your awareness to those sensations in a gentle manner, without self-criticism. We do this to develop greater concentration and train the mind to become our ally. This is called establishing a mind of "single-pointed focus." It is a method to calm the restless "monkey mind."[1]

Sometimes people say that when they try to meditate their mind becomes restless and overactive. The truth is that what they are experiencing is what their mind has been doing all along. They notice this mental busyness only when they sit down and become quiet. Anything that comes up in meditation already exists within us. The development of greater concentration is not about creating new or different thoughts or feelings but rather bringing awareness to our experience in the present moment. The Buddha taught this approach to his followers and was so convinced of its effectiveness that he said, "This is the way for the purification [emotional release] of beings, for the overcoming of sorrow and lamentation [sadness and grieving], for the destruction of suffering and grief."[2]

When we are healing from a loss, an illness, or an accident, our physical, mental, and emotional conditions are likely to become more noticeable to us in the quiet of meditation. We might think that our symptoms have worsened, but again, it is much more plausible that we have simply increased our awareness. Breathe gently and remain calm. If we look for some sort of cure emanating from our meditation practice, we will likely be disappointed. Over time, however, meditation and the insights to which it leads can indeed be transformative.

As an example, if our healing process is filled with concerns about the future—how we will manage, how we will fit in, how people will see us—those thoughts and concerns will arise in

---

[1] "Monkey mind" is a term used in Buddhism, Daoism, and Neo-Confucianism meaning restless, unsettled, confused, wandering, uncontrollable, and so forth.

[2] *Satipatthana Sutta* (Foundations of Mindfulness), Majjhima Nikaya No. 10 and Digha Nikaya No. 22.

our meditation. They draw us away from the present and into the future. Healing and recovery can only happen in the present, as is true of all experience. Meditation has been shown to be a powerful tool for bringing us back to the present moment. It is the essence of the practice. The mind calms, the body eases, medical skills and the human body's miraculous propensity for healing flow most effectively.

Calm allows clarity, from which skillful understanding and wisdom can arise. In meditation, we observe thoughts, feelings, and sensations without clinging to them, pushing them away, or judging them. They are not "my thoughts." They are simply thoughts that arise. There is no possessor of those thoughts, feelings, and emotions; they are not happening to a self. There is only the experience. It is as if to say there are thoughts but not a thinker, feelings but not a feeler, emotions but not an emoter. (A tip of the hat to Mark Epstein, PhD, for his book titled *Thoughts Without a Thinker*, Basic Books, 2013.)

An alternative approach to beginning your meditation session is called a "body sweep." Beginning at the top of the head, move your awareness slowly down through the body. Again, practice without self-criticism. You did not purposefully create stress or tension. Do not punish yourself for noticing it. Slowly scan downward and accept what you observe.

You could also start your session by bringing awareness to sound. There is almost always sound around you. Just hear the sound. It is not necessary to identify its source or name it—car, neighbors, or the like. Notice, if you have preferences, sounds you like and those you dislike, and see if you can let those preferences go, and just hear sound.

Insight meditation focuses on awareness of thoughts, feelings, and sensations, seeing them for what they are—thoughts, feelings, and sensations. As such, they are real, but they should not be accepted as reality. This is seeing things as they truly are and can lead to a sense of peace and equanimity. It is the groundwork for the awakening of wisdom. It is important to note that this does not mean suppressing feelings. Denial of feelings does not move us forward and can lead to a plethora of psychological issues.

With concentration well developed, we learn how to observe whatever thoughts and feelings may arise without adding our story lines to them. For instance, if the thought *I have a meeting today* arises, we simply notice the thought without adding, *I look forward to that meeting*, or *I can't stand those meetings. They're always so annoying.* The reality is there will be a meeting; the rest we are adding on. What we are making up may be based on past experience, but the reality is that there will be a meeting. It is important to know the difference between what is real and what is perception. We do that with straightforward observation.

A creative way to look at thoughts, feelings, and sensations is to envision them as the unexpected visitors in Rūmī's beautiful poem, "The Guest House":[3]

> *You, O human, are a guest house.*
> *Each dawn a new arrival.*
>
> *Be it joyfulness, sadness, or ugliness,*
> *a moment of awareness presents itself*
> *visiting unexpectedly.*

---

[3] Jalāl ad-Dīn Muhammad Rūmī (1207–73) was a Persian poet, Sufi mystic, and theologian.

Make them all feel welcome!
The entire lot of sorry guests,
who impudently vacate your house
of all belongings,
yet, treat each of them as an honored guest.
They may be clearing the way
for some new joy.

Darkness, shame, enmity,
joyfully welcome them into your house.
Let gratitude fill you.
For every one of them has come
from afar to offer guidance.

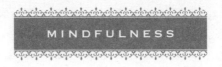

Mindfulness is in. Seminars, workshops, courses, and classes are becoming more ubiquitous every day. The word "mindfulness" is in constant use, although regrettably, the same cannot be said of the practice. The optimistic among us might think that we are becoming a "mindful nation" (to quote Ohio's congressman Tim Ryan). I am among the hopeful, although at this point I can only go so far as to say I think we are *slowly* becoming a more mindful nation. That is progress and I support it with all my heart and energy.

So what exactly is mindfulness, and what does it mean to be a mindful person?

> *Drink your tea slowly and reverently,*
> *as if it is the axis*
> *on which the world earth revolves—*
> *slowly, evenly, without*
> *rushing toward the future;*
> *Live the actual moment.*
> *Only this moment is life.*
>
> —THICH NHAT HANH

From its roots in the Buddhist tradition, mindfulness is viewed as a spiritual or mental practice that is of major significance on the path to awakening. The Pali word for mindfulness is *sati*, which accurately translated means "remember."[1] In actual use, it is about presence of mind and focused awareness on the present without habitual reactions, rather than memory regarding objects or events of the past.[2] The practical relationship of "remember" to "mindfulness" is about remembering where you are and what you are doing. In other words, remembering to be present.

From a pragmatic perspective, mindfulness is about establishing and maintaining a moment-to-moment consciousness of our thoughts, feelings, physical sensations, and surrounding environment. An important element of mindfulness is that we maintain that ongoing awareness, while remaining nonjudgmental. We accept what we notice in our practice without being self-critical. When the mind wanders back into the land of memories or ahead to fantasies of the future, where both our hopes and fears are created, we gently invite our awareness to return to what is happening in that very moment. It does not take long to realize that the real action is in the present. In fact, the only time we can live life is in the present moment.

Although we speak of the practice of mindfulness developing from Buddhist meditation, a secular approach is legitimate and is essentially what is practiced in non-Buddhist American circles. But even a secular approach will inherently have a spiritual quality. An essential element that makes mindfulness what

---

[1] Pali is a Middle Indo–Aryan language of many of the earliest extant Buddhist teachings, as in the Pali Canon.

[2] Buddhist scholar Bhikkhu Bodhi points out that the word *sati* is derived from the verb *sarati*, meaning "to remember," and occasionally in Pali, *sati* is still translated in a way that connects it with the idea of memory. When it is used in relation to meditation, however, we have no word in English that precisely captures its essence. An early translator used the word "mindfulness." This served its purpose admirably and so it has remained.

it is, as opposed to simple awareness, is intention. The mind of a sniper on a rooftop may be intensely focused on his target, and he may be acutely aware of his environment and the tension within his body, but he is not practicing mindfulness. The quality of pure, or wholesome, intention must be present in the practice of mindfulness, and that quality is spiritual in nature.

Meditation and mindfulness each have a significant role to play in our lives, and while there is certainly a relationship between them, they function differently. Meditation can be thought of as the tool that prepares us to live mindfully.

In meditation we first practice concentration during which we gently but adamantly insist that the mind return again and again to a chosen object of concentration. In this part of the practice, we often have to be quite persistent. Concentration can come down to determination. It is usually developed by willpower and patient repetition, and once developed, it can retain some of that determined flavor.

Concentration, properly used, can be of immense value on the path to liberation, but it cannot bring you insight into your self. It cannot see into issues such as greed, anger, and delusion. It cannot penetrate into the nature of suffering. That is the role of Vipassana.

Vipassana, or insight, has a gentler feel leading to awakened discernment. These two, concentration and insight, are the pillars of meditation. *Concentration* provides the stability. It keeps our attention steadily on one object and does the work of holding the attention steadily on that chosen object. *Insight* picks the objects of attention and notices when that attention has gone astray. Insight notices everything that is passing through the mind. There is no such thing as a distraction, because that interruption is observed with the same interest as any other object of meditation. Awareness flows from one object to the next with change itself being observed with interest.

Insight, unlike concentration, is not developed by assertiveness. It grows out of realization, by relinquishing, by practicing easefulness in the moment, and letting yourself get comfortable with whatever arises. This does not mean that insight happens all by itself. Energy is required. Effort is required, but this effort is different in that it has a gentle quality. Insight is cultivated by a softer effort. Persistence and a light touch are the keys. Insight is developed by constantly bringing yourself back to a state of awareness.

Concentration and insight prepare us to live mindfully. With concentration and insight in balance, we are able to bring mindful awareness to our daily activities. Mindfulness in our lives has no inherent limitations. It can be brought to every moment and to every situation that arises. In mindfulness practice, we do not use one object of concentration. Our choices are unlimited and constantly unfolding. We are able to see ourselves as we really are, including any selfishness, greed, and ways in which we cause suffering for ourselves and others. Of course we also gain insight into our most positive qualities as well. We see things as they really are, and in the Buddhist tradition, that is called wisdom.

Mindfulness has no goals. It is just noticing and remaining aware moment to moment. Mindfulness does not create anything. It only observes what is already there. Mindfulness can be practiced no matter what your mood or physical condition. You can move quickly or slowly. You can be energetic or fatigued. You can be shooting a jump shot or stirring the soup. You can be laughing, crying, joyful, or angry. No matter what is going on, you can always be mindful.

Mindfulness is learned slowly, so allow your self to experience the joys of small progress. We all have the ability to be present to our own life and the world around us. We can walk calmly and practice mindfulness of what is happening in the present—mindfulness of the body, mindfulness of the mind, mindfulness of our feelings, mindfulness of all things. By doing this we practice focusing on the present. When a thought arises, instead of allowing it to take us away into a fantasy or a concern, we observe it and gently let it go. We return our awareness to what is happening right now.

Thoughts and feelings are always arising. The purpose of practice is not to get rid of them but to increase our ability to be aware of them. We let things arise naturally and notice them. We bring our awareness gently to them. We might notice our hopes and expectations. Sometimes we look right past what we have in the present because we are looking for something better to happen in the future. Craving for tomorrow cheats us of today. We never really experience life—just desires and fears.

One of my teachers said, "Being mindful is not difficult. Remembering to be mindful is difficult." Living mindfully has been a goal of mine for many years, but during this long period of healing it has been a necessity. It is being present that keeps me grounded. In the moments when I lose that grounding, fear, anxiety, and stress are all ready to step in with their cloying, seductive ways. Fortunately, with practice, we develop a nose that can smell their repugnant presence.

Here is a basic introduction that will help develop mindfulness as a way of living. It is based on the work of my first teacher, the venerable Vietnamese monk Thich Nhat Hanh.

Begin your day with twenty minutes of seated meditation.

There are classes, teachers, and books that can help you get started. See the reference section at the back of this book.

After your meditation session, take a few moments to recall what thoughts or feelings came up most frequently that drew your attention away from your object of concentration. It is not necessary to draw any conclusions. Just take note.

Two or three times each day, stop what you are doing, close your eyes, and bring your attention to the sensations of the next five breaths. Breathe slowly. In the back of your mind you can think, *In, out, one . . . In, out, two . . . In, out, three . . . In, out, four . . . In, out, five.* But your primary focus should be on the sensations of the breath.

Each day, choose an activity that you do regularly and make that an object for practicing mindfulness. One day you may choose to focus on everything that you drink that day—water, juice, tea, coffee, and so forth. Drink slowly and mindfully, noticing the aroma, the taste, the sensations of the liquid in your mouth, on your tongue, and the flow down through your throat.

Another day you may choose brushing your teeth as your object of mindfulness. Slow the process down, especially if you sense that you are rushing. Notice what the toothbrush feels like in your hand and what the toothpaste tastes like in your mouth. Feel the brushing motion and the refreshing sensation. As you drink water or rinse afterward, do that mindfully as well.

On another day you might make the object of mindfulness every door handle you touch. You may be surprised to find out how many doors you open and close each day. Slow down as you touch the handle and bring your awareness to the handle itself. Does it feel smooth or angular? Is it round or is it a lever? Does it feel warm or is it cool? What are the sensations in your hand as you turn the handle? Be specific, and if you find that you have missed a few handles, you can repeat the practice the next day. There is no need to be self-critical.

Each week choose at least one meal to eat in silence. Chew each mouthful of food thirty times before swallowing. This is an eye-opening practice and, yes, it will take longer to eat this meal, so allow extra time and enjoy the treat. To be practical, it might be best to choose a meal that you will be eating by yourself. It makes eating in silence easier and you will not be delaying others.

Let us call this mindfulness practice "The Enjoyment Journal." When you are enjoying a particular event or a specific moment, increase your awareness of your thoughts, feelings, and sensations. Later on, write down if you were actually aware of your feelings while the event was occurring. What were those feelings? What was your mood? What sensations did you notice within your body? What feelings are you experiencing as you write this all down? Be concise and specific while keeping things light.

Living mindfully requires no output of capital, no purchase of equipment, and the most minimal investment of time. It is, without question, the greatest bargain available anywhere on earth. Of course there is a difference between something being available for free and something being given to you. No one can give you mindfulness. To live mindfully requires effort, but the effort can be so worthwhile when the benefits are so abundant. This bargain will always be available but the best time to take advantage of it is now.

GENEROSITY

When newcomers approached the Buddha and asked him to teach them the dharma, he began a series of progressive teachings with the practice of generosity. Commentators have suggested that the reason for this is that without a heart and mind open to the needs of "all beings," the practices of morality, compassion, concentration, and mindfulness—the foundations of Buddhist philosophy—would not find fertile soil. It is important to remember that "all beings" includes one's self, and while dealing with the challenges of healing, a kind and generous spirit directed toward self is essential.

It is an act of generosity not to blame yourself for being in an accident or developing an illness. There is no need to suffer mentally and emotionally. If you focus on intention, you will see that it is highly unlikely that you intended to become ill, get injured, or cause harm. Therefore, blaming yourself is unskillful and only exacerbates stress and turmoil. It is wise to learn from our mistakes but unwise to burden oneself with blame and condemnation.

If beings knew, as I know, the results of giving and sharing,
they would not eat without having given,
nor would the stain of selfishness overcome their minds.
Even if it were their last bite, their last mouthful,
they would not eat without having shared,
if there were someone to receive their gift.
—THE BUDDHA, *Itivuttaka* 26

It might almost seem counterintuitive to think about giving to others when you are the one who is hurting. We are involved in our own suffering and sometimes forget that others are dealing with adversity as well. No one goes through life without experiencing unpleasantness. There is no more effective way to free our mind of our own troubles than by giving to someone else. The smallest token from you can provide a major uplift for both you, the giver, and the recipient. Generosity is the ground for developing compassion. It is not so much about the act of giving as the feeling of wanting to give, of wanting to share. This feeling of wanting to give is considered the heart of a spiritual life. We can also give simply because it feels good, and good feelings are particularly welcome during the healing process. It is a powerful practice to be generous when you are the one feeling in need.

Generosity is characterized by nongreed, nonattachment, compassion, kindness, and joy. For most of us, generosity needs to be practiced and developed because of the underlying allure of attachment and greed. When we develop generosity, the mind becomes freer and more receptive to insight. It is through giving with a loving heart that we develop our capacity to let go.

We learn to give gladly, with respect and with happiness. If our generosity does not bring happiness to our self and to the recipient, we might want to examine our motivations for giving, and perhaps even reevaluate whether we want to give at all.

A gift of value is a gift that can benefit the recipient. In that act of giving, the giver's self-absorption wanes, attachment is diminished, and kindness finds physical expression. According to the Buddha, when one gives with a generous heart, "before giving, while giving, and after giving, the mind of the giver is happier, more peaceful, and uplifted."[1] There is little that could do more for the healing process.

Generosity to oneself can take the form of a sincere commitment to our own well-being. Self-compassion and self-caring balanced with wisdom, help us become the person we want to be in the world. Such commitments require insight and determination in order that we may be able to withstand the physical and mental challenges that can arise within the body and mind. Through meditation or other contemplative practices we can develop a mind of "single-pointed focus." When that level of precise awareness is directed toward a positive goal, we are practicing mindfulness.

Lay Buddhist practitioners—those who practice Buddhist teachings but are not monks or nuns—often commit themselves to living by five basic precepts. These are nondogmatic and can ally with any religion, spirituality, philosophy, or agnosticism and atheism. They guide a way of living that is a great gift to oneself and to the world. These precepts are: to not kill or do any harm in the world; to not take anything that is not freely given; to not engage in sexual misconduct; to not lie or use abusive language; and to not indulge in intoxicants.

By giving up doing any harm, we offer to those around us freedom from fear, hostility, and oppression. By so doing, we ourselves enjoy the gift of freedom from fear, hostility, and oppression.[2] We

---

[1] *Anguttara Nikaya* 6.37.

[2] "There are these five gifts—pristine, of long-standing, traditional, ancient, unadulterated, and respected by the wise. A noble one gives up the destruction of life and abstains from it. By abstaining from the destruction of life, the noble one gives to those around him freedom from fear, hostility, and oppression. By giving to those around him freedom from fear, hostility, and oppression, he himself will enjoy immeasurable freedom from fear, hostility, and oppression. This is the first of the great gifts.

are free of concerns regarding retaliation. The same logic applies to the other four precepts.

There may be times when you just do not want to give: you feel closed off and you cannot rouse even a modicum of compassion. It does not mean that you are a stingy person or have an unkind heart. It may just be a difficult moment. At the next opportunity, see if you can open your heart to yourself and to others. Ultimately, you will be glad that you did. Generosity awakens a sense of well-being. You realize that you have enough to give.

The generosity that was showered on Susanna and me from friends, associates, colleagues, and complete strangers when I returned from the hospital was absolutely overwhelming. During our most difficult times, the openhearted generosity of people lifted our spirits again and again. There was so much joy shared between giver and receiver.

There are many reasons not to be generous, but none of them brings happiness.

"Further, a noble one gives up the taking of what is not given. By abstaining from taking what is not given, the noble one gives to immeasurable beings freedom from fear. . . . This is the second of the great gifts.

"Further, a noble one gives up sexual misconduct and abstains from it. By abstaining from sexual misconduct, the noble one gives to immeasurable beings freedom from fear. . . . This is the third great gift.

"Further, a noble one gives up false speech and abstains from it. By abstaining from false speech, the noble one gives to immeasurable beings freedom from fear. . . . This is the fourth great gift.

"Further, a noble one gives up intoxicants, the basis for negligence, and abstains from them. By abstaining from intoxicants the noble one gives to immeasurable beings freedom from fear, hostility, and oppression. He himself will enjoy immeasurable freedom from fear, hostility, and oppression. This is the fifth great gift."

—*Anguttara Nikaya* (AN 8:39; IV 245–247)

By August 2013, I was walking fairly well but I felt that I was not as steady on my feet as I had been before the accident. So I freed up some precious time and began to study the ancient martial art form of Tai Chi Chuan. I enjoyed my lessons right from the beginning and my balance has markedly improved. There is a legendary claim that Tai Chi can prevent more than six hundred different ailments. The veracity of such a claim is not as important as the actual benefits each individual can experience through the practice. Tai Chi requires a completely focused mind, as does insight meditation. For me, daily practice of both is not only pleasurable but, more important, highly beneficial.

One day my teacher told me that he had mentioned to a friend that I was studying with him. The woman apparently became quite excited, saying that I was one of her heroes because of the way I had fought back and showed no signs of bitterness. I do not see myself as doing anything heroic, but apparently psychologists report that when recovery from trauma becomes overwhelming, people often give up and their lives descend into bitterness. In the accident and its immediate aftermath I fought for my life, which I believe is so instinctive that anyone else would have done the same. Since then I have been striving for as much healing as possible. This may not be as instinctive and has certainly not been an easy row to hoe. For me, the key is often to find joy in the effort.

I try to remember to bring grace, gratitude, and humor to my daily endeavors. I remind myself that my efforts are not so much about overcoming an event in the past, or trying to build a better future, but rather to concentrate on my work and to experience the joys and delights that are right here in the present. I do not try to deny that some days are difficult, but the bigger truth is that I was not expected to live through my injuries, and yet I did. It makes me more committed to doing all the good I can with the time I have left, be it a day, a week, or a decade or two.

Although it is sometimes said that the road to hell is paved with good intentions, I have found that the more challenging the task, the greater the need for intentions—clear, ethical intentions. Buddhists say that our karmic imprint is determined by the intentions that motivate our actions. We often have little or no control over the results of our actions, but we do have control over our intentions. Whether or not we believe in karma is not important; knowing our intention is important. Once our intention is clear, it may have to be backed up by considerable effort. Certainly that will be the case when it comes to recovering from a traumatic event.

Just about everything we do requires effort. Going out for a meal with friends, reading a book, and going to a movie are examples of effort expended on activities most of us enjoy. Even efforts afforded endeavors we do not relish can feel positive if they result in a sense of accomplishment. As the effort eases we can be left with positive feelings, and what was effortful can then seem effortless. This positivity is an antidote to the more anxious feelings that can arise when we must face a challenging undertaking.

Effort is often needed when we decide to address an area of

our lives that is not working well. We recognize that if things are going to change, we have to put in effort. We begin by letting go of the belief that something or someone outside of ourselves is the cause of our unhappiness, and with well-directed effort we strive to see the situation as it really is. Our happiness and unhappiness lie within ourselves. Therefore, that is where our work is to be done.

Moderation is an important part of effort. It helps us know when to work hard, when to rest, and to sense the difference between resting and procrastinating. Without developing effort, we can become disillusioned when faced with new challenges. We must make a conscious decision to apply unwavering energy to our most formidable endeavors. In making such a decision, we are eliminating certain possibilities in favor of other, wiser ones. An hour of work may be more worthwhile than an hour of watching television.

We have surprisingly little control over the world around us, but we do have control over our perception of things. It is in our perceptions that the world becomes either loving, joyful, and peaceful or harsh, unfriendly, and fearful. Often when we have to do something that is new for us and it does not come easily, we can become frustrated and anxious and we want to quit. When a new challenge seems likely to test our intellect, resolve, or courage, we are often tempted to back away in order to protect our self-image and not damage our delicate ego.

Focus on effort, not results. When we see life as an ongoing process—a process that includes challenges as well as easy times—we can accept the fact that some things simply require greater effort. There is nothing wrong; it is just the nature of things.

Another effective form of introspective practice that I use daily is called *metta*, or Lovingkindness Meditation. There is a charming legend that tells of its origin. It seems that the Buddha, sensing that certain monks were ready to advance in their practice, sent them to reside and practice meditation for the rainy season in a nearby forest. Soon after their arrival they were "assailed by tree sprites" who were annoyed by their presence. The sprites created terrifying sounds and disgusting smells, causing the monks to become frightened, lose their concentration, and flee the forest.

They hurried back to inform the Buddha of their experience. The Buddha instructed them, "There is no other resting place that is right for you. It is only by living there that you might reach the end of taints and stains. So go again and occupy that same resting place. But if you want to be free from the fear of sprites, then learn this safeguard, for this will be both protection and a meditation subject for you." He then taught them the *Karaniya Metta* discourse.

The monks returned to the forest chanting the words they had just learned. The tree sprites were so charmed by the now unflappable monks that they sat quietly and listened, and never again did they upset the monks.

THE PRACTICE of metta has the potential to become a healing and liberating presence in one's life. The benefits of this meditation become clearer the more one practices it. Metta is uplifting, loving, and compassionate and trains the mind to be more kind and generous of spirit. It helps cultivate our natural inclination for an open and loving heart. It is a structured and specific practice in which we offer thoughts of lovingkindness to ourselves and to all beings. For those actively involved in healing from a traumatic event, offering kind and loving thoughts to one's self can be a soothing balm. For all of us it is a deterrent to the belief that we are, in some way, unworthy. Contemplating the goodness within ourselves is a classic practice that awakens the joy within. Metta practice is not about increasing egoistic tendencies. It is a commitment to our own happiness, understanding that our happiness is the ground for developing a love for all beings.

Metta practice begins by offering silent thoughts of lovingkindness to oneself, then to someone who has been particularly good to us, for whom we feel gratitude and respect. This person is traditionally known as a "benefactor." Then we move to a loving friend, but not one who has been or is a sexual partner. It is usually relatively easy to direct lovingkindness to these beings (we say "beings" rather than "people" to include those of the animal kingdom).

Next we move on to those for whom it may be more challenging to offer metta. In doing so we have an opportunity to widen our vision and expand our capacity for kindheartedness. We call the next recipient of our metta a "neutral" person. This is someone with whom we may cross paths often but about whom we know little, such as the letter carrier, the person who sells us our newspaper each day, a neighbor, and so forth. Then we move on to a "difficult" person. This is someone we are not getting along with at the moment, or perhaps with whom we have never gotten along. If this is a new practice for you, do not start with your worst enemy. Someone with whom you are mildly annoyed is fine for openers. With practice, the "enemy" will be easier. Finally, we offer lovingkindness to all beings. No one should be excluded, including those we do not particularly like.

Through this practice we can cultivate friendly, loving feelings for ourselves and for all beings. During the practice we do not try to make any particular feeling happen. We observe different feelings as they arise at various times. It is our intention that is most important. We are planting seeds, and seeds bear fruit in their own time.

To practice, find a place to sit that is quiet and where you will not be disturbed for fifteen to twenty minutes. Repeat the phrases in your mind at a pace that allows you to maintain concentration. The phrases you use should be comfortable for you, so feel free to modify these words:

May I be safe.

May I be happy.

May I be healthy.

May I live with ease.

(To "live with ease" refers to dealing with life's everyday activities—relationships, children, traffic, the workplace, and so forth.)

Next, envision and offer metta to a benefactor (sometimes described as one who brings a smile to your face): *May you be safe; may you be happy; may you be healthy; may you live with ease.*

Next, envision and offer metta to a close friend: *May you be safe . . . etc.*

Next, envision and offer metta to a neutral person—someone for whom you have no strong feelings of like or dislike: *May you be safe . . . etc.*

Next, envision and offer metta to someone with whom you are having difficulty: *May you be safe . . . etc.*

Next, offer metta to an ever-widening circle—anyone in the room with you: *May you be safe . . . etc.* in the city, the state, the country, the earth, the universe, the cosmos, those no longer living, those not yet born: *May you be safe; may you be happy; may you be healthy; may you live with ease.*

Repeat the phrases and then allow a period of several minutes of silence. You can conclude your practice by reading the Metta Sutta before moving mindfully into your next activity.

THE KARANIYA METTA SUTTA

This is what's done by one skilled in what's good,
Who reaches toward that most peaceful state:
One would be capable, and straight—quite straight;
Well-spoken, gentle, without too much pride;
Content with little, easily maintained,
Not doing too much and lightly engaged;
Thoughtful, with a peaceful demeanor, and
Modest, without greed among worldly things.
One would not do even the slightest thing
That others who are wise would speak against.
May they be secure and profoundly well;
—May all beings be happy in themselves.
Whatsoever living beings exist,
Without exception, whether weak or strong,
Whether tall and large, middle-sized, or short,
Whether very subtle or very gross,
Whether visible or invisible,
Dwelling far away or not far away,
Whether born already or not yet born

—May all beings be happy in themselves.
Let no one work to undo another.
Let no one think badly of anyone.
Either with anger or with violent thoughts,
One would not wish suffering on others,
Just as a mother would watch over her
Son—her one and only son—with her life,
In just the same way develop a mind
Unbounded toward all living creatures.
Develop a mind of lovingkindness
Unbounded toward the entire world:
Above and below and all the way 'round,
With no holding back, no loathing, no foe.
Standing, walking, sitting or lying down,
As long as one is devoid of torpor,
One would resolve upon this mindfulness
—This is known as sublime abiding here.
Without falling into mistaken views,
Endowed with insight and integrity,
Guiding away greed for sensual things,
One would not be born again in a womb.[1]

Throughout the day, at any time, try looking at anyone with whom you cross paths and silently offer them metta: *May you be happy.* When in traffic or waiting in line at the market, even when in a disagreement: *May you be happy.* When you are alone with your aches and pains, your anger or sadness, offer yourself

---

[1] In this translation, American scholar Andrew Olendzki strictly observes the original meter of ten syllables per line. He also stays with the original male reference "son" rather than the more universal "child." Sometimes translators have to make difficult choices.

a sincere moment of lovingkindness: *May I be happy.* It is an entirely different way of being in the world. Try it and see what it feels like.

THE LOVE offered in metta is pure, without any sort of agenda or possessiveness. The love offered by friends that has supported Susanna and me through our ordeal has had that element of purity beyond what I ever could have imagined. I have now experienced in real life that the greatest gift we can give to one another is our presence. That means being entirely there for the other with no desire to advise, fix, or entertain. This type of presence arises from a purity of love for the other person, not a sense of obligation or feeling of responsibility.

My friend Natalie lost her husband in the tragic events of 9/11. She spoke often of the extraordinary love offered to her by family, friends, and complete strangers. That love remains strong in her heart even as the sadness continues to recede. I too find that the details of my accident fade, but the love that has supported Susanna and me feels more present than ever. I am alive because Susanna's love was strong enough and determined enough to face down all those professional medical opinions.

Ultimately, love cannot conquer all, but it makes the journey worthwhile. I think the secret is not to seek love but to offer love. It is not always easy to find the best in each person—that which is loving and lovable. Some seem intent on hiding their most beautiful attributes. Keep trying. They need you and you need them.

Freedom and love go together.
Love is not a reaction.
If I love you because you love me, that is a mere trade,

a thing to be bought in the market;
it is not love.
To love is not to ask anything in return,
not even to feel that you are giving something—
and it is only such love that can know freedom.[2]

---

[2] From *Think on These Things* by J. Krishnamurti (1895–1986), who was born in Mandanapalle, India.

CONTINGENCIES

I am sometimes asked how I have remained free from bitterness in the wake of such a terrifying and debilitating accident. Although it was never my purpose to prepare specifically for an airplane crash, I believe that many of the practices I have worked with through the years stood me in good stead. They helped me stay grounded not only in the chaos and urgency of the crash itself but also in the dark days that followed.

I do not devote energy to questions like "Why me?" or "How could this happen?" I can never know the answers to such queries beyond an understanding of what is known as "dependent origination" or "contingencies." This view of natural order is an understanding of life in which we see that everything is interconnected. Nothing exists separately; nothing just drops out of the sky (including the plane I was in). Everything is affected by everything else and everything arises (or falls) due to specific causes and conditions. The traditional language in Buddhist texts states it this way:

> *When there is this, there is also that.*
> *With the arising of this, that also arises.*
> *When this is not, that is not.*
> *With the cessation of this, there is the cessation of that.*

Everything that is, is as it is because other things are. A pilot brought a plane down short of a runway. The plane, flying low, cut through electrical wires and sparked a fire that engulfed the plane. The plane crashed. I tried to jump from the plane but my foot got caught on something and I was seriously burned before I could free myself. My mind/body immediately went into survival mode and I did survive. That is what happened. A great deal of physical, mental, and emotional pain has been involved, but in terms of what happened, that is it. It is what we call the "bare experience." It is free from the infinite number of story lines, projections, and perceptions we can attach to such an event. It contains no regrets, accusations, or blame. It allows the road to recovery to be unencumbered.

The Buddhist teachings focus on understanding the nature of things as they are, rather than speculating about what might have been if things had been different, or what might happen in the future. I never looked back speculating about the possibilities if I had not flown that day. I never screamed or yelled although I shed a few tears. I never blamed the pilot, the airline company, the Burmese people, or a God. I never wearied myself with the burden of anger. Even if I were to say, "I wish I had not been on that plane," I would have had to be someplace, and who knows what might have happened in that other place?

Sometimes when a terrible event happens, we say, "He was in the wrong place at the wrong time." What we rarely, if ever, think about is how often we have been in the *right* place at the *right* time. We do not think about how many times a driver stopped her car when the light was turning yellow rather than speeding up and going through. Consequently, we were not hit by a car. We do not think about how many times we were not hit by a stray bullet, or how many planes we were in that did not crash. It is said that the Angel of Death walks beside us. The message is not to live in fear but to be present to every moment.

The doctrine of dependent origination helps us understand that we are part of a complex web of events, most of which are out of our control. Acceptance eases our journey.

Sure, I would rather not have been in that crash, but I have never been able to foretell the future. So I relinquish any hope for the past to have been different and I focus instead on the present. The present is the only time we can experience all the joys, beauty, and delights life has to offer. It is also the only time we can focus on healing. I do not want to miss out because of stumbling around in the darkness of the past.

As to the "Why me?" question, the most logical answer is "Why not me?" Bad things, horrible things, happen to people every day. That just happened to be my day. Who am I to be exempt? My task now, my responsibility to myself and my loved ones, and my opportunities all center around my ability to heal, and that is where I am directing my energy.

When we look closely and fully grasp the law of dependent origination, we see that our lives are not a series of arbitrary events. Conditions are continuously unfolding, bringing about the events of each specific moment. When we see the truth of dependent origination, we then see that we are not helpless or powerless. We are constantly making decisions that affect the course of our lives. When we understand how things happen, we also understand how to create change. We create change by changing conditions, not by trying to change results. It becomes our choice to create conditions that lead to different results and greater happiness for ourselves and for others.

We have surprisingly little control over the events in our life, and certainly we cannot change events that have already happened. We can, however, change how we relate to those events. In other words, we may not be able to prevent an illness that has invaded our body or injuries resulting from an accident, but we do have control over our perceptions, our understanding, how we experience those events.

We must understand and accept what *cannot* be changed. My hands will not function better because I wish them to do so. They will function better because every day I meticulously do the exercises I have been taught. They will function better because of the work ethic I bring to them. My hands are heroic. They were seriously injured but they are fighting back. They will again throw a ball, autograph a book, and eat sushi with chopsticks. They do not know what it is to quit. They will prevail.

Illnesses, injuries, loss of a loved one, loss of employment, and the ending of a relationship are among life's most difficult challenges. Who among us is not familiar with these forms of dukkha? The common cold, the noisy neighbor, the arrogant colleague at work, the stiff back, the setback, and the headache are forms of ever occurring dukkha. The range of dukkha is limitless and its nature is profound.

Dukkha is actually a characteristic of life interwoven with its joys and pleasures. A "characteristic" is an element or quality inextricably connected to something else and can offer insight into the nature of that other thing. Heat is a characteristic of fire because when there is fire there is heat. A characteristic is not necessarily good or bad, it simply is. When we understand that difficult times are as much a part of life as joyful times, we can accept life's challenges with greater ease and a sense of equanimity. It does not mean that loss, illness, and injury are enjoyable. It simply means that they are a part of life and we all have to deal with them.

I believe that one reason my recovery has gone well is that I do not muddle the healing process with unanswerable questions. With the clarity offered by dependent origination, I do not have to ponder whether or not I did something wrong by getting on that plane, or if I was being punished in some way. I am not burdened with either guilt or the need to blame. My job is to heal while at the same time living life as the person I want to be.

Anger

Anger is an acid that can do more harm to the vessel
in which it is stored than to anything on which it is poured.
—MARK TWAIN

Anger is a normal emotion usually related to our view of having been treated unfairly, wrongly, or in some way denied something to which we feel entitled. It can also involve a powerful emotional response to a perceived provocation and include a desire to retaliate. The presence of anger may be accompanied by increases in blood pressure, heart rate, and levels of adrenaline. Some research indicates that anger is a factor in our fight-or-flight response.[1] Anger is rarely beneficial, usually feels uncomfortable, and often lays the ground for unskillful and even dangerous actions. Signs of anger that are not always recognized as such include threats, blaming, refusing to forgive, manic behavior, obsessiveness, bullying, and selfishness. If we have been fortunate enough to enjoy excellent health throughout our life, we can feel indignant or disgruntled when even a mild cold invades our body and slows us down for a few days.

[1] W. Harris, C. D. Schoenfeld, P. W. Gwynne, A. M. Weissler, "Circulatory and Humoral Responses to Fear and Anger," *The Physiologist* 7 (1964), 155.

The Buddhist view of anger:

An angry person looks unattractive and does not sleep well. When he gains a profit, he turns it into a loss by doing damage with word and deed. A person with anger destroys his wealth. Maddened with anger, he destroys his reputation. Family, friends, and colleagues shun him. Anger costs him dearly. Anger inflames the mind. He does not realize that this danger is created within himself. An angry person does not know the Dharma [Truth]. A man overcome by anger is as if blind. He takes pleasure in unskillful actions as if they were good, but then, when his anger subsides, he suffers as if burned by fire. He is spoiled, obliterated, as if enveloped in smoke. When a man becomes angry, he has no shame, he does not fear evil, and is not respectful with his words. For a person overcome with anger, nothing brings joy.[2]

The Dalai Lama adds, "If we live our lives continually motivated by anger and hatred, even our physical health deteriorates." It is pretty easy to check this out for yourself. When you find you are in the throes of anger, stop for a moment; look within and see if you feel comfortable. Notice how there is no peace or joy when anger is present. This is a particularly detrimental state for one whose mind needs to be focused on healing.

The work involved in diffusing anger is not about denying its presence. It is about developing greater insight into the destructive facets of this potentially dangerous emotion and then

---

[2] *Kodhana Sutta*, Anguttara Nikaya 7.60.

mindfully releasing its hold on us. Although anger can do damage throughout the body, its origin is in the mind. It is your mind; you are in charge and your mind can be trained to become your greatest ally. For some, the guidance of a trained psychotherapist or participation in an anger management program might be advisable. For others, the wisdom to see the need to change might be motivation enough.

No one is just "an angry person." That is too simplistic for such complex creatures as we are. We have a vast array of emotions arising and fading away constantly. We want to pay particular attention to anger because of its potential destructiveness and our susceptibility to anger while dealing with trauma, illness, or injury.

Here is an exercise that can be quite effective. It is a bit more sophisticated than the basic "count to ten" practices and can yield profound results with minimal but sincere effort. When anger arises we tend to think, *I am angry*, by which we are characterizing ourselves based on a feeling. There is also a false sense of ownership of that feeling. Instead, try backing away to get a more spacious view, as if you were looking through binoculars turned the "wrong" way. Then bring awareness to what you are feeling as you think, *There is anger arising. Sam* [use your name] *is experiencing anger. Isn't that interesting. . . . Sam is now experiencing intense anger. . . . Wow, there is a sense of rage. . . . The anger seems to have a reddish color. . . . It really is quite interesting. . . . Now the anger seems to be subsiding and Sam is feeling more peaceful.*

It may take a bit of practice so that this exercise does not feel contrived, but the results have great potential. It requires that you take the time to look beyond the surface to the deeper levels of your experience. After a while the "Sam" fades and you see that there is no self that has to be protected, defended, or aggrandized. There is no self that is being threatened, only your perception of self.

Our life can be transformed by even a minimal change in our perceptions. In other words, we can control our experience of life. While the arising of anger may be a natural phenomenon, there is no need to act out based on that feeling.

There is little that can cause anger to arise as quickly as pain. Psychologists tell us that pain, anger, and depression are often experienced as one massive, often overwhelming emotion. They caution that when we do not differentiate among the three, they can end up reinforcing one another. When I was young, I often acted out with anger because I did not understand, or could not accept, that what I was really feeling was sadness, or hurt, or fear. It was a great relief, when in therapy, I worked my way through to the truth.

The eighth-century Indian scholar and philosopher Acharya (Teacher) Shantideva warned that just one moment of anger could destroy the good that we have accumulated over many eons. He asserted that anger, like no other force, leads to suffering, grief, sadness, and despair. He also contended, however, that once we see the uselessness of holding on to our anger we are well on our way to overcoming it. The courageous act of starting to address our anger could truly be referred to as noble and life changing.

We know that we do not enjoy pain, but what most of us never explore is the complex nature of pain. So, we know nothing about pain other than we do not like it. Emotions play a significant role in the experience of pain, and pain births anger. The helpless feeling that can be brought on by an illness, accident, or loss can make anger seem appealing. It has energy; it is active, it helps us feel alive and invigorated. It feels so much better than sadness. We must, therefore, be mindful, because while anger is a perfectly normal emotion, acting on anger is rarely beneficial and, in fact, is likely to have serious and lasting repercussions.

The energy of anger is powerful. We feel it throughout our body. The chest pounds, the head spins, and the gut churns. But anger often comes upon us in a surreptitious and treacherous manner. It seduces us by journeying through the ego and creating a false sense of purpose. We feel stimulated and motivated, and if there is anything that is appealing when we feel down and out, it is motivation. We may not notice the subtle desire to have others feel our pain. The nurse disturbs us, so we strike out at him. *Someone should pay for the pain I am feeling. Surely someone is at fault.*

We can adamantly cling to our anger without an awareness of the hurt we are causing our selves and others. We need wisdom and patience to overcome the powerful energy of anger and irritability. With wisdom, we see that anger is an emotion. It is not something that is embedded in us. Although the current vernacular uses the term "hardwired," neuroscientists are not suggesting that there is a part of us that is immutable. Rather, they are saying that we are born with certain characteristics and propensities that are sometimes associated with "personality." That does not mean that such characteristics are rigid and fixed. Today's research shows that not only can we change, but we are in fact in a continuous state of change. Therefore, it makes sense to use the characteristic of change, or impermanence, to our advantage. It is not an exaggeration to say that to disengage the "buttons" that trigger our anger could save a life—perhaps our own.

Too often we experience an emotion and then attach to it as if it were an innate aspect of our very being. You might believe that you are "an angry person," ignoring that the basic nature of sentient beings is more likely compassionate and kind, not angry and unpleasant. We need to understand that anger is not a part of who we are but rather that it is a feeling that arises with certain causes and conditions. It is called a "conditioned phenomena." Like anything else that arises, feelings pass away. They do not define character.

Repeated outbursts of anger most likely indicate the presence of fear and unhappiness. They are unpleasant to experience for you and those around you, but they are not fixed, permanent conditions. Again, it is important to remember that even if we frequently experience the arising of anger, it does not define who we are. There is nothing to defend. With practices like mindfulness, meditation, compassion, and lovingkindness, we can transform our anger into more positive, productive energy. When anger, resentment, bitterness, and other such feelings take hold of us, we cannot enjoy peace of mind. Anger can seem to have value, but look carefully. There might be some logic to responding with anger if it could change what has happened, but it cannot. What has happened has happened, and we can only move forward.

Regrettably, we must acknowledge that many women may have a difficult time when it comes to transforming anger. As a culture we have a history of raising our female children to be "the peacemakers." Even though we live in a more enlightened time, the remnants of such thinking still remain. It is fortunate that women tend to be highly sensitive beings and, generally speaking, more attuned to their feelings. That is the key to overcoming the destructive power of anger for both genders. We start with awareness. We learn to recognize the feeling of anger as it arises, and then we mindfully create a pause between that feeling and any ensuing actions. Here is a valuable hint: As soon as you sense the feeling of anger within you, shift your attention quickly and mindfully away from what you think is the source of the anger and focus on your feelings. That is how you create a pause in which you can consider what would be your wisest option.

If this is a new concept for you, be aware that there may be years of conditioning and habit energy pulling you in the direction of an angry reaction. Ego makes anger appealing. You must have clear intentions and determination to overcome its allure. It is important to understand that this practice is about being mindful of anger, not suppressing it. Suppression does not free us of anger and will likely create its own psychological issues. Observe and acknowledge your anger. The feeling is perfectly normal. Understanding the destructive nature of anger yet not acting on it is wisdom.

The causes of anger are many. One example is a sense that we have not been treated fairly. "Why has this happened to me?" we ask. If on any level we cling to a belief that life should be fair, it is we who are not treating ourselves fairly. Life unfolds as it does and fairness is not part of the equation. If I seek an answer to the question of why I was injured in a plane crash, then I must also inquire as to why I did not die as the doctors said I would. Both questions are worthy of investigation but then must be accepted as unanswerable.

The practice of acceptance helps us to undermine anger. That makes it possible to not just survive but to thrive.

COURAGE

You gain strength, courage, and confidence by every experience
in which you really stop to look fear in the face.
You are able to say to yourself,
"I lived through this horror. I can take the next
thing that comes along."

—ELEANOR ROOSEVELT

Relinquishing control of our world and accepting that things just *seem* to happen makes life a lot more tolerable, even though some of the things that happen may not be pleasant. Accepting that an illness has invaded our body or that an accident has left us injured and incapacitated can be challenging. When a trusted friend has betrayed us or a loved one has been unfaithful, we can be left reeling and devastated. Yet without the burden of trying to change everything around us, free of figuring out who or what to blame, and released from the dismal task of vengeance, we are available to direct our energies to the more productive task of healing.

No matter what practices and/or exercises one has mastered—be they spiritual or secular—there are likely to be moments when we will simply have to be brave. Physical pain can be excruciating, mental anguish can be consuming, and emotional turmoil can be torturous. In the fourth act of Giacomo Puccini's romantic opera, *La Bohème*, Rodolfo has just realized that his beloved Mimi has died. His close friend Marcello cries out compassionately, *"Coraggio!"* which, in that highly emotional moment, hardly needs translation.

Courage is a mental factor. Therefore, developing this valorous quality is a matter of mind training. It might seem as if courage could be developed only in real-life situations where courage is required. Even if that were the case, there are times when just getting out of bed can require courage. Proposing to one's beloved, asking for a raise, and buying a house all require courage. Depending on the individual and the given circumstances, any action might require a degree of courage.

We can also develop courage on the warm and welcoming meditation cushion. One time we were planning an African safari that required taking several small aircraft flights between camps. I had done this comfortably on previous safaris so there should have been no cause for concern. But one morning I woke up with a chilling sense of fear that I would be claustrophobic on the small planes. I had never experienced claustrophobia nor was I experiencing it at that moment, but rather I was feeling a fear of claustrophobia. Since claustrophobia is itself a fear (of confined spaces), I was actually experiencing a fear of a fear. The fear was so overwhelming that within minutes I became convinced that I could not go on that trip. Then I realized that this whole experience was in my mind. I sat down, closed my eyes, and envisioned myself in one of those tiny aircraft. I allowed the fear to arise and it was indeed powerful, but I continued to see myself in the plane with the fear until it subsided a bit.

I did the same exercise again that evening and again the fear subsided somewhat. The next day I did the exercise again, and by the end of that day the fear was gone. As it turned out, the safari was fantastic and it would have been a shame to miss it. This way of "rehearsing" allows us to practice courage in a safe environment. Familiarity with a situation helps us to feel more comfortable.

I have been going on meditation retreats for years and I seem to always have the same experience at check-in time. I arrive in a cheerful mood, breathe in the country air, greet friends, look over the schedule for the week, and head for my little room. Once I am inside the room, an apprehensive, almost panicky feeling begins. I have no idea why, and after all these years I have let go of my desire to understand why. The feeling always fades away by the time I have made up my bed. Although the retreat usually does not begin officially until after a light evening meal, I have had my first opportunity to practice observing the arising and fading away of emotions. I have come to enjoy that awkward time because it allows me to feel that I am getting a head start on the actual retreat.

Facing fear head-on takes away its power, pries open its fingers, loosens its grip from around our throat, and reveals it for what it is—a feeling. Like the mist that rises from the river on a cool country morning, it fades away to the land of memories. It has no legs to go the distance. It has only the energy that we provide. We can look directly at our fears and say, "I know you, you are a feeling. You can stay for a cup of tea but I am going to have dinner without you."

A serious injury or illness can alter one's physical appearance. We can be left with a scarred body, a demolished psyche, a limp, a lump, a loss of limb, diminished mobility, and any number of other reminders of the fragility of human existence. Learning to adjust physically, mentally, and emotionally can be a major undertaking.

For me it often takes courage on a daily basis as I work my way back from the plane crash to the life I want. Part of that process involves accepting that there are things that I will not be able to do as I had done them before. In a very real sense it takes courage not to cling to the past but to be with the realities of the present. Otherwise it would be so much more difficult to make the adjustments necessary to again have a meaningful life.

Courage is not fearlessness. It is being willing to acknowledge and face our fears and uncertainties even if they are daunting. Physical courage is the willingness to face pain, and even the threat of death. Moral courage is the willingness to do what is right even though popular opinion sees things differently. Sometimes it takes courage just to breathe in the next breath.

FRIENDS I

The first few weeks after the plane crash, doctors in Myanmar, Bangkok, Singapore, and New York all painted a grim picture. Simply stated, they felt I could not survive my injuries. Once I had met Dr. Tan and then Dr. Yurt, both of whom felt I could return to full function, their optimistic prognosis took over and became a beacon brightly lighting my way. There were still doctors who said I would not make it, and there was still considerable pain and struggle with which to deal, but I believed "full function" was in my future.

Then one day while on my way to one of my various therapeutic appointments, I noticed an attractive middle-aged woman in a wheelchair. I wondered if her future included "full function," and if not, how did that affect her healing journey? What if she had been told, "You will not walk again"? And what about those who have been told that they have a terminal illness? What might their journey be like? Would they be able to heal even if they could not be cured?

Jennifer

(Please note that this chapter contains graphic descriptions of violence.)

Jennifer was born in Chicago in 1960 and moved to Phoenix, Arizona, in 1998. Prior to her injury nine years earlier, she was a massage therapist with a corporate business background. She enjoyed her work, which she felt gave her the opportunity to do something that was meaningful with her life. She wanted people to be glad to see her and to benefit from her efforts.

> JENNIFER: I'm a mom and adore my son. At the time of my injury, he was twelve years old. I was divorced, and engaged to the man who was injured with me. I had a very busy, active, and happy life. I felt fully realized as a human being, understanding of course that there is always plenty of room for growth. I was in the present without worrying about the past or the future. Looking back, I suppose there was a bit of arrogance in me, perhaps even overconfidence.

Jennifer and her fiancé, David, had been on vacation in Fiji for two weeks, scuba diving and relaxing. Their first night back, November 15, 2004, they worked teaching martial arts classes until 10:30. (Jennifer has three black belts.)

> It was a perfect night. We were completely relaxed, rested, feeling that nothing could get us down. We were incredibly happy. In Fiji, David, after numerous previous attempts, had asked me again to marry him, and this time I finally said *yes*. Back home that night we drove to get something to eat because we were too jet-lagged to prepare a meal at home. We pulled into a little Mexican drive-through restaurant that we liked and a vehicle pulled up next to us on the driver's side.
> Suddenly, from out of nowhere, the driver fired five

shots at us. We were startled by the loud sound and we both started to get out of our car. I thought, *What the hell just happened?* I opened my door and put my foot out and David said in the calmest voice, "Get down." I didn't understand what was going on. The shots were incredibly loud and I know I was screaming; I was screaming profanities. I grabbed my cell phone and tried to call 911 but I couldn't get a signal.

The shooting stopped and David sat up intending to drive away and escape. But then there were two more shots. David's words now went from clear, intelligible speech to gibberish, just sounds. Then he slumped over the steering wheel. The last bullet (a third) hit me in the back. It was like a hot electric jolt going through my body.

Our car kept going forward and hit a tree, deploying the air bags. It became very hot inside the car. The horn was blaring and there was so much going on. It was so hot inside the car that I couldn't breathe. I wanted to open the door to let air in but I didn't want the shooter to know I was alive.

Then suddenly the door on David's side opened and I was certain there was about to be a bullet in my head. But it was a passerby who stopped to help. He started talking to me and I was also able to get through to 911.

I was immediately paralyzed by the shot. In the days following my injury I found that the bedrock of my beliefs was shaken. I now had no idea of what reality was.

With an oxygen mask over her face Jennifer was rushed to the hospital. Every person who came along, whether in the ambulance or in the hospital, she grabbed and pleaded with them to tell her son how much she loved him. (The shooting took place nine years earlier and Jennifer had told her story many, many times, but whenever she spoke to me about her son, her voice trembled and she cried.)

The whole time—from the moment she was shot, the ambulance ride, and being taken into the hospital—she felt an overwhelming love; love for her son, for her fiancé, for her community. That connection made her sad because she was certain she was going to die. At the same time, there was also a fierceness stemming from her refusal to leave her son.

> I think there are times when we actually make a decision about whether we will let go or whether we will fight to stay alive. Each time I closed my eyes and started to drift, it was my love for my son that made me open my eyes again.

The first hours in the hospital were chaotic. Countless people were asking so many questions, but still what mattered most to Jennifer was that someone tell her son how much she loved him. Then, hours later, they finally brought her son, Matt, to see her.

> It was late at night so he had been asleep, and when I saw him he looked so small, and pale, and disheveled, and so scared. He was trying so hard to be brave. It is when I recall that moment that the mom in me hurts the most. I know it wasn't my fault, but I felt that I was

the cause of my son's suffering. To this day that still hurts me deeply.

She described the next three or four weeks of her existence as being like a TV medical drama. All through this time there was no question in her mind that she was going to die. Added to that was the fact that the doctors were not saying anything to alleviate her fear.

Parts of both of her lungs were removed; ribs were wired together, and she was put into a medically induced coma to heal. When she woke up, one thing she really wanted was a shower. A friend had taken her hair down and began to brush it out. It was matted with blood, bone, and bits of brain matter. They were brushing pieces of her fiancé's brain out of her hair.

I asked Jennifer what it was like to be lying in a hospital bed all that time certain she was going to die.

My mind kept coming back to my son with thoughts like *Why didn't I spend more time with him?* Then there were thoughts of things like *Who's going to feed my dog? How will people know where to find this key or those records?* All of those dumb things would pass through my mind but always I kept coming back to how much I loved that child. There was a great deal of physical pain, but the emotional pain was much worse.

I wonder if my son would be more whole today if he had been hit with the entire trauma all at once and I had died that night, instead of being subjected to the ongoing traumas of my situation. I'm just not sure if it was the best thing. It's a matter of all the additional trauma that has come these nine years as a result of my having survived with a severe disability. So many times he and I have rushed to the hospital with the real possibility that this was the day his mom was going to die.

For nine years all this ongoing trauma and constant struggle has been on my child. So sometimes I wonder which would have been the better world for him to heal in. I'm in the middle of another health crisis even right now as we speak. I'm always dealing with what to tell him and when to tell him. I don't want him to think I'm withholding information from him. I don't always know if survival was best.

I'm not a believer in "God saved you for a reason; you are here for a purpose." I am here and I am creating a purpose for myself. I am an activist. I am willing to take the risks. I am already broken; what else can happen to me? I feel I have nothing left to lose. I am capable of speaking up and advocating for issues. So I feel that the purpose I have created for myself is to make life better for those who come after me. I am an advocate for those who may not have the skills or ability to speak up for themselves. That's my focal point and role.

Jennifer said that with all the interviews she had done related to the crime, she had been asked so many times about the details of the shooting and her injuries, but never before had she been asked about her feelings around it. It was a new and challenging experience. I felt grateful that she was willing to explore this with me. She replied:

Emotion this intense with so much sorrow is never fun. It's an interesting experience and I'm sure I'll be exploring it for many days, and probably longer. This is like suddenly looking over the edge and realizing how far down it is. So I'm going to step over the edge, let go, and see what happens.

Her first stay in the hospital was for five months.

I felt extremely isolated during that time. I had very few visitors, partially because of the extent of my injuries and also because the police carefully monitored anyone on my floor. I quickly became a news story, with the media constantly coming around looking for new angles, new ways to keep the story going. I had constant pain and I lived with an ever-present awareness of mortality. There was also the ongoing process of gaining back my strength and learning how to use my body.

It took a few weeks just to learn how to sit. For a while I could not sit up at more than a 30-degree angle. I took all of my meals lying down. The first super effort I made was learning how to sit. There was no longer any muscle strength to support my head and shoulders. It probably took as much effort to learn how to sit as it would take for someone to learn to walk on a high wire. I had to learn how to remove my physical waste from my body since I no longer had any internal control. I had to learn how to use a catheter and I had to learn how to remove my feces from my body. I had to learn how and when to do these things. The enormity of what it means to live inside a paralyzed body is absolutely overwhelming.

ALLAN: Did you ever have any feeling of being less of a person, or of being less human than those around you?

JENNIFER: Oh, yes, absolutely. I would turn militant. *I am no less of a person than you. I will show you.* I still struggle with that. I often feel invisible, and when I am visible, I'm seen in the stereotypical way. While I am now internally quite comfortable with who and what I am, the activist in me very much fights against the stereotypes. *You will treat my community with respect, with openness, with awareness. I'll teach you to do that by requiring that you do it with me.*

ALLAN: Do you get belligerent?

JENNIFER: Yes, sometimes.

ALLAN: When I was in the hospital, I cried often enough that they sent someone from the psych department who decided I needed to be on medication. What about you? Did you go through depths of sadness?

JENNIFER: I cried often. I also explored with the hospital staff, who were essentially my only visitors, the difference between grief and depression. Once I left the ICU and got to the neuro-acute unit, they pretty much had a protocol for how they dealt with people like me. It involved a social worker who came to check on me every day. We would talk about the future and what we were going to do with me; where I would go for rehabilitation and then where I would go to live, because I was going to lose the home that I owned.

Every day she would come into my room and every day before she left, she would try to get me to say, "I am permanently paralyzed." Obviously I needed to accept my injury. I certainly knew that I was paralyzed and that was not going to resolve itself in any way. There wouldn't be a treatment, a drug, or a microchip that would make it all better. The social worker was annoyed because I refused to say what she wanted me to say. "I have a spinal cord injury. I am paralyzed. There is no known cure." It made her insane that I refused to say I am permanently paralyzed. I just couldn't get there with her. Certainly my situation was very bad. I had been shot in the back and I was paralyzed.

At one point Jennifer was moved to a different unit within the hospital and there was confusion with her paperwork. As a result, she went for a long period of time with no pain medication.

I'm not a wimp. I've given birth, broken bones, and plenty more, but this pain was intense. In order to deal with the severe pain, I began examining the specific nature of the pain itself. I referred to this as "directing my mindfulness to the pain." I allowed the pain to be inside my body without being afraid of it. I even eliminated the word "pain" and just allowed it to be my current sensation. I am not a fan of pain and I assure you I would much rather live without it, and yet, strange as this may sound, there was something exquisite about the experience. It involved letting go of the fear and the labels and just letting it be. It became a practice of just observing sensations and I found it interesting.

What Jennifer did was change her relation to the pain. She could not take the pain away but changing her relation to, and perception of, the pain totally changed her experience.

Her situation was enormously difficult; so many questions had to be faced. Where would she live; how would she live; what about the needs of her child; what would her insurance cover; and on and on. At the hospital, they recommended an antidepressant and Jennifer again asked what the difference was between grief and depression. She questioned the wisdom of medicating grief, which she saw as very real and appropriate at that time. She did not agree with the idea of "muting her grief." Would she then not have to deal with it sometime in the future?

It was a major event to get from her hospital bed to her wheelchair. She cannot cough, so she chokes easily. It now takes two hours to get out of bed, showered, and dressed rather than the previous twenty minutes.

> I dealt with a great deal of fear and anger, and at times I still do. For me, a healthy emotional state now involves a certain level of tension. I can rouse considerable self-pity. Society encourages me to do so. I could give in to helplessness; I could give in to despair. I don't know if I'm going to be alive to see Christmas. [It was December 5.] I could give in to any of those feelings, but I choose not to, which sometimes requires a discipline of not allowing myself to go there. As you said, Allan, it means not spending time with unanswerable questions.

I asked Jennifer how society encourages her self-pity.

> When I'm in the supermarket, people move out of my way with a certain look that says, *Oh my God, that could be me.* People speak to me in a different tone, the kind of tone they use with a lost child, a voice that's a little higher, a little sweeter, a little breathier. They change the words that they use so that they use small, simple words.

I'm not the most gregarious person. I prefer my solitude, which I think is usually obvious. I'm not in any way soliciting conversation with strangers. Yet complete strangers will approach me and say, "It's good to see you out." Someone might come up to me, pat me on the shoulder, and say, *Bless you*. If I were my former six-feet-tall, athletic self, those are interactions that people would not be having with me. Sometimes they offer me a concerned, "May I help you with that?" I won't allow people to pity me. That would create a tiny existence for me.

Overall I am happy, content with my life. There still are areas of grief and stress I want to release. I suffered tremendous loss. My fiancé, David, is alive but we cannot be together. He requires 24-hour-a-day care and I am not able to give that. The conflicting nature of our ongoing needs makes it impossible, which alone is an enormous loss. Yet overall, maybe happy is not the right word, but I like who I am and I like my life. I like where I'm going although there are places where I'm very dissatisfied. But the fact that I'm paralyzed doesn't leave me paralyzed with grief.

I thought about a time when I heard the Dalai Lama say that if you read about the circumstances of his life, you would likely say that it has been quite a difficult existence. He was forced to leave his homeland and his people more than fifty years ago and has never been allowed to return. He has not succeeded at what is so important to him, specifically, negotiating an acceptable existence for the people of Tibet, and he has had health issues. Yet he said, "I am happy."

The perpetrator has never been caught. For a long time Jennifer often thought about how much she wanted justice. She wanted the shooter to pay for what he did. Ultimately, however, she was able to free herself from the shackles of a vengeful mind. She believes that by trying to gain vengeance, one just gets caught in an ugly cycle that does not change anything. Even if the "bad guy" were caught, she still would not be able to walk. This type of realization was instrumental in helping Jennifer move forward.

> I experience joy. My life is not a living hell. Sometimes when people feel comfortable enough with me to be truthful, they have said that if what happened to me had happened to them, they could not live with it. They would have killed themselves.
>
> My experience is that the human default is not just to survive but to thrive. We are not fragile. We are strong and we are tenacious. We move forward. I think sometimes it takes more effort to stay stuck. I think that fear is the great limiter. I'm not saying that I have overcome fear. I do many things fearfully, breathlessly. The extent of my injury has given me courage. My body is broken but my spirit is whole. I think my spirit has become much more fierce.
>
> There are things I would like. I would like more comfort, I would like less pain, I would like more convenience, I would like many things, but I have a good life. I am happy with who and what I am.

Jennifer is an avid user of Facebook. Here is an entry from her page on December 2, 2013:

Tomorrow, December 3, is International Day of Persons with Disabilities. This year's focus is *Break Barriers, Open Doors: for an inclusive society and development for all.* I ask you each to spend tomorrow being mindful of the barriers to inclusion in your surroundings—both physical barriers as well as policies and attitudes. One in three people in the USA is disabled. Everyone is a heartbeat away from the illness or injury that could add you to this, the least exclusive club on the planet. Within every person lie unique talents and abilities. What door will you open? What barrier will you eradicate? Who will you include?

The mutual friend who introduced me to Jennifer advised, "She is a force." That was not an exaggeration. I found Jennifer to be bright, articulate, and direct. She uses her abilities to help those who cannot help themselves.

Stephen

I met Stephen early in 2013 when he began coming to the Community Meditation Center. He never had religious or spiritual interests unless one counts the fact that he practically viewed George Harrison of the Beatles as his spiritual guru.

Thirty years earlier, as a young man of twenty-three, he was attending chiropractic school in Minnesota when an arteriovenous malformation was discovered in his spine.[3] The condition left him completely paralyzed from the chest down.

---

[3] Arteriovenous malformation (AVM) is a defect of the circulatory system. An AVM can develop in different areas of the body, but those located in the brain or spinal cord can have especially widespread effects.

The day I became aware of the paralysis moving upward from my legs to my midsection to my chest, I knew enough about anatomy from my chiropractic studies to realize that if the paralysis continued moving upward and got to my neck, it would kill me. That night I was preparing myself to die. As I recall now, thirty years later, I kept my composure. I was quiet, not "freaking out." I was not indifferent to the circumstance, but if I was going to die that night I wanted to be aware of what was happening at that most important time. I wanted to be "awake for the show."

I was taken by ambulance to the nearest hospital emergency room. The ER staff didn't know what to make of my situation. The doctor on call telephoned a neurologist who, based on the information given to him on the phone, offered a diagnosis saying that I most likely had multiple sclerosis. He decided that he did not need to come in to see me. After a surgical procedure the next day, the doctor told me that everything now seemed normal. So I never received an official pronouncement of "you will never walk again."

For the first few weeks, I would wake up each morning thinking this was a dream, very vivid, but nevertheless a dream. I was living with unreal hopes. It was some time before the "foreverness" settled upon me. I recall having a few moments when I broke down, but mostly my memory is of being upbeat. As a young person, my experience of illness was always that it would pass. You would be sick for a few days and then you would be better. The news of the situation was much more serious, and it took time to let in the reality. It became harder to cling to the notion that it was just a dream.

Learning bladder and bowel care was a major challenge. I no longer had any control over my bladder or bowels. This was the greatest source of shame and embarrassment. Everyone around you is focused on the fact that you can't walk, but I adjusted to that more easily. The psychological side was devastating and mortifying.

Stephen had bladder accidents all the time, causing him to live with constant anxiety. Because of this he wanted to stay close to home. As the realization of his paralysis set in, over the course of time he went through a period of despondency, grief, and hopelessness. As we discussed what had unfolded thirty years ago, Stephen spoke of these things with a certain ease.

At one point he read Stephen and Ondrea Levine's book, *Who Dies?* He identified with it closely because, in a very real sense, he felt that he had died. His peers at that time were advancing in their lives and careers, becoming doctors, lawyers, and Wall Street brokers. He felt extremely unaccomplished, and the comparisons were painful.

Stephen has been meditating on and off since the 1980s and feels it has served him well, but mostly he has learned from paralysis. "There is no way to get around it," he said. "Paralysis is a big teacher."

At one point I decided to seek counseling with a psychologist. During our initial sessions I remember describing to her that I felt as though I had "lost my personality." I couldn't locate my sense of humor, which had always been so accessible. Though I never succumbed to clinical depression, I was feeling depressed just the same. With her help, I developed an insight to the fleeting nature of these brief spells of depression and learned to take a mindful step back and observe how they burn themselves off like a fever. This has been a particularly profound and enduring lesson for me. Gradually, my "lost personality" came back; it had never really gone away, of course, just obscured by cloud cover. The sense of wholeness that I had been searching for was slowly restored, annealed by the therapeutic process of self-examination and discovery. And I felt myself again deserving of being loved.

Stephen grapples with nihilism.

This life is it. There is nothing more. When you're done, you're done. If there were a miracle cure, that cure would be, for me, a trauma in itself. I spent all this time reinventing myself, carving out a new identity, and now I'm cured? I would be back to being some everyday jerk on the street. What happened to all the hard work that allowed me to stand out from the crowd? I can be this someone who could be admired, while coping and adjusting. But that was a young person's blood. Metaphorically I had died and then I was born again, and had to go through childhood and adolescence. In adolescence you are very self-conscious. That is no longer true.

My interview with Stephen took place almost a year after my accident. As I looked over my notes and reflected on our time together, I was struck by what seemed to be an incredible ease with which he handled the first year of his incapacitation. There was a matter-of-fact, casual manner as he spoke, which was also present in a short autobiography he had written many years ago. I wondered if Stephen had been forthcoming about what he was feeling in that first year. Even when acknowledging sadness, it was couched in phrases like, "I developed an insight into the fleeting nature of these brief spells of depression" or "my 'lost personality' came back; it had never really gone away, of course, just obscured by cloud cover." He seemed so comfortable, while I still struggled.

Then came the obvious yet profound insight: There is no one way to heal; there is no one best way. The best way is the way that works for the individual, and it is likely to be different for each of us. We can learn from one another. We can support one another, but ultimately it is for each of us to take the steps that create our path, the path to wholeness.

Rather than offering Jennifer's intensity, Stephen is rarely without a smile on his face and a humorous comment on his lips. Two people, two paths, two ways of accepting, two whole individuals.

FAITH

The dictionary tells us that "faith" is a noun, but actual life experience reveals that faith would be more accurately described as a verb. According to the *Oxford English Dictionary*, a noun is a word "used to identify any of a class of people, places, or things," while a verb "is used to describe an action, state, or occurrence." Viewed as a quality of life, faith, like patience, is not a thing that can be possessed or lost, nor is it solid and unchangeable. Faith develops as we see things more clearly, and that clarity, or the ability to see things as they really are, is wisdom. So we see that there is a deep connection between faith and wisdom.

When perceived as a verb, we would think of ourselves as "faithing" rather than "having faith." From the Buddhist perspective, there are three stages of faith, the first being "bright faith." In this stage, we experience something that touches or moves us. It attracts us, or uplifts us. It may be a book, a philosophy, a teacher, or anything that inspires us—it begins to open our eyes. But whatever it is, it is someone else's truth until we try it for ourselves by living it.

Thus, the next stage is called "verified faith." This is where we probe, question, and investigate, seeking clarity in order that our budding faith might become substantiated. This is necessary for our faith to evolve into "enduring faith" (sometimes referred to as "abiding faith"). At this level, we do not "have faith" but rather we and our faith are deeply connected and are as one.

In the days and weeks following the events of 9/11, I was fortunate enough to be able to serve the families of victims as well as many of the volunteers who came to New York to assist. Reports afterward told of large numbers of clergy who, in the face of such suffering, resigned their posts. Many of them lost faith in their previously held beliefs. Accounts revealed that most of these clergy had accepted their beliefs since childhood with blind faith that had not been substantiated through their own experience. The horrors they saw at Ground Zero, as well as the widespread profound suffering, unraveled that faith to the point where it could not be sustained.

It is a wise practice to examine what we so readily accept as truth, or what we believe because we have always believed it, or what we "know is true" because it is what we were taught. A serious loss, illness, or injury can shake our beliefs unless they are well grounded. There is no reason to fear this type of self-inquiry because if our beliefs are established in truth, investigation will serve to verify that truth. There is no reason to believe that misfortune has occurred because we are being punished. There is no way to verify such thinking. Things happen, some of which we find pleasant and some of which we find unpleasant. That is verifiable by looking back at our own history and the history of those around us. It is the way things are. No one goes through life without adversity.

If we observe our own body, we will see how it does everything that it can to heal itself. Sometimes there is no cure for our illness but the body does all that it can to bring us to the most advantageous state of health possible. We seek the best professional advice. We employ technologies, methodologies, and medications to help the process along. We strive for the utmost clarity and calm in our thinking in order to allow the body to function in as stress-free a manner as possible. The miraculous human body, even when struggling, will verify the faith we have in it.

THINKING

A man is walking home late one night when he sees his friend Mullah Nasrudin down on his hands and knees under a street light. "Mullah, what are you doing?" the friend asks. "I'm searching for the key to my house," Mullah replies with agitation. "I'll help you look," the friend says as he gets down and joins Nasrudin in the search. Now both men are down on their hands and knees looking for the key.

After considerable time searching in vain, the man asks Nasrudin, "Tell me, Mullah, do you remember where you dropped the key?" Nasrudin points back toward his house and says, "Over there, in my house. I lost the key inside my house." Now annoyed and confused, the friend jumps up and shouts at Nasrudin, "Then why are you searching for the key out here in the street?" Nasrudin answers, "Because there is more light here than in my house."

So many of us seem to be searching for a key. We may be seeking the key to happiness, or the key to liberation, or to inner peace, or to good health—all of which are worthwhile pursuits. We believe that the key is in wealth, or power, or relationships. That is where the light seems to be. We have lost sight of the fact that the key lies within; it always has, it always will. But the search must be made in the darkness of our fears and insecurities. Artificial light does not work within. The key can only be found where it resides, not where it is convenient to look.

There is a short series of teachings of the Buddha that collectively is called the *Dhammapada*. In Sanskrit, *Dhamma*, in its broadest sense, refers to all truth or reality. *Pada* means "path." Together, we have "The Path to the Truth." In Christianity, it is said that if all the teachings that were offered by Jesus were lost, and we had only the Sermon on the Mount, we would have the essence of all of Christianity. In Buddhism, we could say the same about the *Dhammapada*. If the thousands of the Buddha's discourses were lost and we had only the *Dhammapada*, these 423 concise verses would preserve for us the essential core of what the Buddha taught. We might even go so far as to say that if we had only the first chapter, we would have enough guidance to create a path for ourselves that would lead to enlightenment; to awakening; to peace and happiness. It begins: "All that we are is the result of what we have thought. It is founded on our thoughts. It is made up of our thoughts. If one speaks or acts with an evil thought, pain follows one, as the wheel follows the foot of the ox that draws the wagon."[4]

This verse has a twin that goes this way: "All that we are is the result of what we have thought. It is founded on our thoughts. It is made up of our thoughts. If one speaks or acts with a pure thought, happiness follows one, like a shadow that never leaves." See the image of the ox drawing the wagon and see that the wheel has no choice but to follow the footsteps of the ox. In the same way, all experience is preceded by thought, led by thought, made by thought.

HERE IS a short story that has been popular in India for many centuries: A man is selected to go to a foreign land to learn about the people. The man is high-minded, kind, and generous. Another man is also selected to go to a foreign land to learn about its people. This man is rather mean-spirited, grumpy, and grouchy. When the first man returns, he reports that he found the people in the foreign land to be kind, gracious, and warm, "very much like the people here," he said. When the other man returned, he reported that he found the people in the foreign land he visited to be mean-spirited and grumpy, not very caring at all, "kind of like the people here," he said. Both men had been sent to the same land.

Two men go to a foreign land. What do they see, what is

---

[4] The term "evil" in this context refers to thoughts, words, or actions that create dukkha, as in the next paragraph where "pure thought" refers to thoughts that alleviate dukkha.

their experience? What they come home with is the creation of their minds. We have all kinds of thoughts throughout the day, and some of them we may not like. The mind is indiscriminate in the creation of thoughts. We do not know why or how thoughts come to be. We do not know where a thought comes from or where it goes, but we can learn to differentiate between which thoughts will lead to suffering and which will alleviate it.

It is most important to understand the difference between "awareness" and "denial." If the thought arises, *I could just strangle Jen for what she said*, we may not like that we are having such a thought. We might like to believe that we are above such thinking. Yet the reality is, we are experiencing an angry, aggressive thought. Denial is unhealthy and ineffective. Then again, if we accept within our self that we are having such a thought, we can look at that thought with awareness, realizing that it is just a thought. With awareness comes the realization that there is no need whatsoever to act upon that, or any thought. Specifically, it would be best not to strangle Jen.

The *Dhammapada* acknowledges the arising of impure thoughts but advises that we do not speak or act while experiencing such thinking. When we see injustice or abuse and we believe we can help, we want to be certain that we are acting with pure thoughts. We want to have a clear understanding of our motivations. If we are aware of our thoughts and motivations, we have a much better chance of acting effectively.

WHEN I first came home from the hospital, all I could think about was how miserable I felt and how desperately I wanted my life back. It was very difficult to focus at that time, which made meditation onerous. It took time and patience, but gradually I was able to return to my practice. Correspondingly, I began to accept the way my new life was unfolding. I lost interest in trying to cling to that which I could no longer do. I would either get those skills back or I would not. In that transition, my new life became more meaningful, dynamic, and deeply satisfying. I will always be grateful for all the wonderful people and experiences in my pre-accident life, but the truth is I seem to appreciate my post-accident life more deeply.

There are always thoughts arising. They arise and they pass away, constantly, one after another, on and on. The Twin Verses are telling us that we have options as to how we respond to our thoughts. Early on in our practice, it may not feel that way because impure or even "evil" thoughts seem adamant about reappearing again and again. The Buddha described this as the nature of the untrained mind. His prescription was the practice of insight meditation. This requires that we take the time to stop; that we give ourselves permission to stop and learn how advantageous it is to stop. Stop the busyness and just be present. You have always been a human *doing*. Now you are invited to be a human *being*.

Sit down for a minute, or five, or maybe twenty or thirty. You might even go on a retreat. For whatever period of time, begin to experience stopping, and in that time take a look within, not judgmentally, but with interest and curiosity. Learn what you can about what goes on in the mind. One thing that we begin to see is that every conscious moment, every thought, every feeling, every aspiration, every intention, is a moment of practice. It is creating a path and it is a moment of practice whether we like it or not. The mind will go where it has become conditioned to go. Condition the mind with dignity and care.

In this practice we take the time to observe, to notice. It does not take long before we see that some thoughts bring about emotions that feel better than others. It does not take long to see that if we follow certain thoughts, we are more likely to be creating a path for ourselves that simply feels happier and healthier. We may notice that we are becoming more patient and more compassionate with our self and with others. The Buddha said it took him ten thousand lifetimes. You may only be on your 174th. You remind yourself that this is a practice. It is ongoing. It is not about arriving at a destination. It is about where you are right now. Then one day you notice that you just handled a situation better than you would have a year ago. This is an important moment on your journey.

We become present to what it is to be alive. We feel healthy no matter what our ailment. It happens in the mind; all that we are arises with our thoughts. Observe those thoughts. If they are not thoughts that advance your cause, say, *Okay, I don't have to go with that thought. It was nice having you visit me, thought, but you are just a thought. Go on your way now.*

Take a look at what is happening in the mind: the likes, the dislikes, the craving for more, the desire for less. Develop insight so that you sense the kind of thinking that will lead to suffering and the kind of thinking that alleviates suffering. When we change our thoughts, we change ourselves. It is not an exaggeration to say that we can change the quality of our entire life.

FITNESS

After two months of hospitals, surgeries, and procedures, I finally returned to my own home. As mentioned earlier, I was barely in the door when I found myself irresistibly drawn to the exercise bike and was able to churn away on it for a few minutes. Physical fitness can be somewhat addictive. The fact that I had to bike slowly and could not last very long, plus having to be helped off when finished, did not diminish the pleasure.

Throughout my entire adult life, I have stayed in good shape because of being committed to a fairly vigorous, and essentially enjoyable, workout routine. Combining that with a healthy diet and the good fortune to have been born with excellent genes, I have lived my life essentially illness free. I was never a body-builder, just in good shape. I have no doubt that being physically fit was a major contributing factor in my surviving the plane crash and the ensuing injuries incurred while trapped in a roar-ing fire. Then suddenly, as if overnight, I was emaciated, too weak to turn on my electric toothbrush, and even when I re-learned how to walk, precariously unsteady on my feet. (I could not even take out the garbage at night, depriving me of one of the American male's most traditional and treasured responsi-bilities.) The body loses muscle tone quickly, but fortunately it also has an extraordinary capacity to rebuild, albeit slowly.

The addition of practicing Tai Chi Chuan[5] was a perfect fit for me and I recommend it highly for anyone who can walk. Since Tai Chi involves slow movements, and complete concen-tration, it could be an ideal practice for someone recovering from an illness or injury (depending, of course, on any physi-cal limitations involved). After an injury, all physical exercise should be discussed with a medical professional and/or your physical therapist. Starting out slowly and easily is always advis-able, and an experienced teacher should be able to adjust a pro-gram for you.

---

[5] Tai Chi is the abbreviation for Tai Chi Chuan, translated as "The Supreme Ultimate Boxing System."

My ankles were particularly injured in the accident. The burns went all the way through to the bone in a number of places and each leg required three separate grafting procedures. Any movement that involved the ankles was uncomfortable, and it seemed as if it was going to remain so. One day, about four months into my Tai Chi practice, I suddenly noticed that my ankles were moving much more freely. The Tai Chi form involves considerable use of the feet, legs, and ankles, and while I have no way of knowing for sure, I feel quite certain that Tai Chi played an important role in this part of my recovery.

My teacher, Dr. Lawrence Galante, describes Tai Chi this way:

> It is an ancient Chinese exercise consisting of slow, relaxed movements for total self-development. For the body it is an exercise. For the mind it is a study in concentration, willpower, and visualization. For the spirit, it is a system of meditation. Tai Chi is also a preventative and curative branch of Chinese medicine and the Supreme Ultimate system of martial art. Once learned, this form can be performed in approximately nine minutes. It is the perfect exercise for today's busy lifestyles and can be tailored to suit individual needs. When performed at a rapid pace with low stances, the form becomes a more aerobic exercise for the heart. Performed very slowly, the stances build muscle tone in the calves, thighs, and arms, and increase bone density.

A friend told me she never meditated because she couldn't think about nothing.

I told her I think about nothing very often, and I think nothing of it.

The idea that meditation is about thinking of nothing is a popular misconception. The practice is, in truth, quite the opposite. It begins with sharpening one's thought process so that the mind and its ability to focus become an ally. As one's mind becomes more focused, the practice moves toward gaining greater insight and the development of wisdom. Ultimately, the goal of meditation is enlightenment, sometimes referred to as awakening or self-realization. Tai Chi, with its emphasis on physical and mental relaxation, partners beautifully with the classic approach to meditation.

Tai Chi Chuan theory and practice evolved in accordance with Chinese philosophical principles, particularly those of Taoism. Since the widespread promotion of Tai Chi Chuan's health benefits in the early twentieth century, it has developed an international following among people with little or no interest in the martial arts, but rather for its beneficial contributions to a healthy mind and body. Medical studies support Tai Chi's effectiveness as an exercise and a form of physical and mental therapy. Specifically, it is suggested that focusing the mind solely on the movements of the form helps to bring about a state of mental calm and clarity. In the last twenty-five years or so, Tai Chi classes that emphasize health benefits have sprung up in hospitals, clinics, and community and senior centers. This has likely come about as the form's reputation as a low-stress training method has become better known.

We can easily fall into the trap of focusing on what we cannot do that we previously could, either because of an affliction or advancing age. It is more productive to be grateful for what we can do and build slowly from there. I began light workouts a few days after returning home but had little stamina and not much strength. I found myself more shocked by my weakness than discouraged. Even on my worst days I managed to push on because I am so aware of the benefits of physical conditioning. Also, to be honest, I did not like the scrawny wreck I saw in the mirror. Sometimes an overactive ego can work in our favor.

By about eight months after the accident, I had returned to my former workout routine, which, in addition to the exercise bike, includes working with free weights and lots of stretching. I do not attempt to work with particularly heavy weights, since at this point full recovery and maintenance are still my goals. I find moderate weights to be effective for those purposes. My body weight is coming back and my Tai Chi practice gives me a lift on many levels every day.

I spend a lot of time, probably too much so, at my desk writing, studying, and preparing teachings. Too many days were going by without my getting outside even for a short stroll. I knew it was an important part of my recovery, both physically and mentally, so I decided to do something about it. I enjoy photography, so I replaced my camera that was lost in the crash and started going to the park with it every day, even if was only for a half hour. Fresh air, a good walk, and some darn good pictures are now part of my therapy.

There is an endless variety of physical exercises in which one can participate, from gentle walking to vigorous boxing. With minimal effort, anyone should be able to create a routine that is pleasurable and effective. The important thing is to be active at some point every day if at all possible. If you are in the process of healing, let the Buddha's teaching of the Middle Way be your guide.[6] Exercise energetically but at the same time, do not overdo it. Listen to your body. It is wise.

FRIENDS 2

Jeffrey

There was an article in the *New York Times* about a man in the Midwest who had built his own coffin. The article said that he saw it as an opportunity to create something of beauty and purpose that would be both a celebration of life and an acceptance of his death. I had an immediate sense that I wanted to speak with this man and so I sought him out.

Jeff is a physician who lives in Kansas. He is married and has four children. Eleven years ago, at the age of fifty-four, he was diagnosed with incurable Stage IV prostate cancer. As Jeff tells it:

> I was very involved in my career doing, oddly enough, mostly cancer surgery, which is about 80 percent of what thoracic surgery is. I was busy and very content with what I was doing and I felt I was doing a good job. Then a routine insurance physical in the year 2001 showed an elevated PSA [prostate-specific antigen]. Although I didn't have any symptoms, I did have a sort of ominous feeling about it. Early in 2002, I had a biopsy

---

[6] The term "The Middle Way" was introduced in the *Dhammacakkappavattana Sutra*, which was the first discourse delivered by the Buddha after his awakening. The Middle Way is a path of moderation between the extremes of indulgence and self-mortification.

that was positive for prostate cancer. The feeling was that we had caught it early.

As part of my job, I had to tell more people than I can possibly remember that they had cancer. I knew from that experience that 80 to 90 percent of the time when people hear the word "cancer," the first thing that comes to their mind is "death." That was not the case with me. I was certainly crushed and this was something that I didn't want to hear, but I felt we could just deal with it—we could tend to it and it would be done.

At the same time, Jeff's mind was reeling. Prostate cancer was not his area of expertise. To whom should he turn? To whom should he speak? Suddenly he had to deal with the same questions we nonmedical people have to face.

Jeff called his wife, Jean, right away and gave her the news. There was a stunned silence on the phone. The next day he called a urologist friend, who responded optimistically, saying that it was probably confined and recommended that at his age Jeff should have surgery. If the cancer was confined, removing the prostate would essentially allow Jeff to get on with his life.

Of course, the big problems with removing the prostate are the possibilities of incontinence and impotence. I was concerned about both. Jean and I met with a urologist I had worked with a number of times and he seemed the ideal person to perform the surgery. He said that the percentage of people who had to deal with either incontinence or impotence was quite small.

Then, because I had spent a lot of time at the Mayo

Clinic, we decided to go up there and get another opinion. I saw a urologist up there who specialized in prostate cancer and he essentially said all the same things. Then he said that he would like to examine me. Within seconds after starting the exam he said, "Whoever told you that this cancer is early on doesn't know what he's talking about. This is a good-size tumor. It can still be removed, but then we'll have to see."

Jeff and Jean made the six-hour drive home and were absolutely devastated. They did not know what to say to each other. This was so much more overwhelming than they had been led to believe. There was nothing more they could do except go ahead with the surgery. They felt crushed, as if they were getting into "the black hole of cancer." While not afraid of the surgery itself, Jeff was quite apprehensive about what was going to be found.

The surgery went fine, but Jeff was distressed to find that he had been left with positive margins in several places.

Simply stated, the cancer had spread. The surgeon tried to play that down, saying that it didn't necessarily mean anything, but frankly I didn't believe him and I was really discouraged.

I wore a catheter for two weeks and went back to work wearing a leg bag. I felt tired but I was all right. The PSA went to zero, which is what you want, because if you have no prostate there should be no PSA reading. I had essentially no problems with incontinence, but I have been totally impotent from that moment on, and that was extremely difficult to accept.

Jeff pretty much adjusted to his new life. Every few months he had another PSA test. Then, just about one year after the surgery, he had a PSA test and when he called in for the results, he was told that it was 0.2. He asked again, and again he was told 0.2. As a physician he knew that was really bad, and sitting there at his desk he had what he described as a "panic attack."

I knew exactly what that meant, that there was cancer still in me, it was growing, and it was not good. I hung up the phone and sat there at my desk. I literally was panicked. The urologist suggested as a next step to have the prostate bed radiated. They explained the possible side effects, which were not pleasant, but I went ahead and had radiation for about three weeks.

Radiation doesn't hurt, but I found it to be a very unsettling experience. In fact, I found it absolutely horrible. There was a voice within me wanting me to just tear off the sheets and run away. You're not just fighting cancer; you're fighting this awful feeling. The side effects, however, weren't bad, and any that I had I got over pretty quickly.

My PSA went down, but then in six months it started going up again. Then I knew for sure what was going on. I knew it was not curable. No one could say how long I had to live and, as we used to say in medical school, "life is an incurable condition." On a certain level I could accept it, and at the same time, I was very angry.

Jeff spoke with his urologist, who suggested that he take a very aggressive approach, starting with taking a medication that would diminish the formation of testosterone. (Prostate cancer is fed by testosterone.) At this time, he read an article about the type of treatment he was receiving, which said that the mean survival after this treatment was about one year. He read that sentence over and over again and realized that he had thought that this treatment would hold back the cancer indefinitely. More research revealed to Jeff that after a while the tumor figures out how to make its own testosterone. That was "panic moment number two."

Then he went on an even more aggressive regime of medication and began what Jeff called "life with an oncologist." There were all kinds of side effects, some mild, some stressful, and some surreal, as if they were happening to someone else's body. He would be on chemo and then off so his body could rest, and then back on chemo again. That regime went on for years, in fact up to the present. In 2005, Jeff retired from surgery because the chemo left his hands numb.

> At that point, I tried to take control of anything that I could. Cancer takes away all control. It is a complete mutiny of the body. You try in any way that you can to get control of any bit of it. You realize that you have the lion by the tail, but you look for anything you can get. I had many different types of treatment, all of which could give me a few more months, but the bottom line was my cancer is incurable.
>
> I've had more than fifty chemotherapy infusions; I've had treatments that required resuscitation. I've been hospitalized twice, once with a high fever that no one could figure out. I've had every antibiotic in the book. I would stare at the ceiling in the hospital room

and think, *Shit, am I going to die in here?* I developed a child-like fear of the night because it was at night that my fever came.

This whole process has brought my wife and me infinitely closer. It has led me to an absolutely unique and beautiful relationship with my children and deepened relationships with my friends. When I was in the hospital and the nights were so difficult, these friends worked out a schedule so that one of them could be with me every night. I had never had such love shown to me. This has all brought so many blessings to my life.

About three years ago, we found a metastasis in my hip. Now we were not just dealing with a number. We radiated that one and it went away, but about six months later we did another scan and there were at least thirty lesions. In 2012, they started me on a drug that was experimental at the time. It was given to me on a "compassionate protocol."[7] You don't ever want to find yourself on a "compassionate protocol," but that's where I was. That drug was effective for a while but now my cancer has spread enormously and there is hardly a bone in my body that doesn't have cancer.

In the last two months my PSA has grown rather astronomically, and now, just in the last three or four days, I have started a new drug that was approved last fall. It's not curative but it might get me a few months.

---

[7] As I understand it, compassionate protocol can occur when a program is full, but because a particular patient is doing very poorly, they make a compassionate exception and allow him in.

But clearly we are running out of time. I never asked my doctor, "How much time do I have?" I know that no one knows, but we all know that the endgame is close.

I asked Jeff if he followed any particular religious or spiritual path. He answered by saying that it was always easier when he had to give bad news to a religious person, but that was not him. He has always had a fairly contentious relationship with the "greater power." When he was dealing with his angry response to his cancer, he went through what he referred to as a rather narcissistic reflex: *Why me? What have I done? Haven't I done a great deal of good in my life?*

Having said that, there are parts of the creative side, a beautiful force that I have absolutely embraced throughout my life. When you do open-heart surgery, you stop the heart. Then you do the work. Then there is a certain maneuver you do to get the heart to start up again. You sit there and watch the heart slowly start. Then it starts to do something purposeful and in a few moments it comes back to a full demonstration of life, beating away. After twenty-five years of doing open-heart surgery, I never got over the wonder of that moment.

If you look around the oncology suite and see people basically all dying of cancer, there is something in their eyes that we don't see in the average person on the street. I think when people really confront death and have at least some acceptance of it, there is the realization that throughout our lives we have accumulated so much stupid baggage.

We were born with a certain kind of innocence. We are given a knapsack and we add things to it—jealousy, anger, greed, grudges, and whatever. What people with cancer understand is how futile it is to carry that knapsack anymore. When you put that sack down, you find yourself in a totally different place. That's where I am.

I can forget grudges. I have sought people out and asked for forgiveness for things I did in the past. I don't want anything except time with the people I love. Without that knapsack, I now listen to the birds, check out what's going on in the trees, talk to strangers, and I am feeling their grace. People ask me if you have to be dying to do that. Well, we're all dying. You don't have to have death staring you in the face, but you do have to accept the fact that you are going to die. That's what this coffin project was about.

There is something fundamentally beautiful in this world, a spiritual force of some sort. To be clear, I do not believe that when I die I am going to some place that is paved in gold and that I will see all of my old relatives. It doesn't fit with my scientific inclinations. But if you ask me if there is a force of beauty in the world that I can address when I'm walking around and be grateful for, and that is giving me something every moment, the answer is yes.

The process of approaching my death has brought me much closer to the person I've always wanted to be.

Abby

Almost at the same time as Jeff's article appeared in the *Times*, there was a letter to the editor from a college professor at John

Jay College of Criminal Justice. Abby was writing about the "How long do I have?" question that almost always comes up when one receives bad news from a doctor. Her insights intrigued me and I decided to seek her out.

Abby is a fifty-three-year-old New Yorker who, aside from her teaching, is a published author, wife, mother of two, and dedicated "gym rat." We met on a Sunday afternoon at a studio she rents to see her psychotherapy clients as part of her work as a college professor.

A few years ago she had a herniated disk and assumed that the pain she was experiencing at the beginning of 2013 was an exacerbation of that condition. The doctors agreed. The pain was becoming quite intense, but she was particularly busy with work, and so she just kept going.

In June, she was walking home from her office and her left leg suddenly gave out. Although she was only a couple of blocks from home, it took her more than an hour to finish the walk. She went back to her doctor and then consulted other doctors.

All they wanted to do was prescribe painkillers. I didn't want to take painkillers but I had to do something because of the intense pain. I started working with a physical therapist, who said that she did not think the pain was emanating from my back as had been suggested by the doctors. She recommended that I get an MRI of my hip.

The doctor performed a complete clinical examination and said that he didn't think the problem was with my hip, but he gave me a script for an MRI. The MRI revealed that, basically, my entire pelvis on the right-hand side had been eaten away by tumors, and my glute was only partially attached.[8] At that point, I knew I had cancer.

I had to get a biopsy. In this town you have to know somebody to get a biopsy [laughs]. I had to wait ten days, which were probably the longest ten days of my life.

The technician who did the MRI said to me that he had never seen a scan like this. He couldn't believe that I wasn't screaming with pain. I was hospitalized right away to get the pain under control.

A few days later, the doctor came in, accompanied by his interns. He told Abby that it was a terminal diagnosis. He asked her if she knew what "terminal" meant. She said yes. The trained psychologist part of her wondered why the doctor had not said something like, "I have news for you. Would you like to have someone here with you?" She thought the protocol was strange. She also was surprised that they presented a terminal diagnosis in front of a group of interns without asking her permission. Did he not realize how devastating that news would be? At the same time, she realized that all her defenses were up so that she could deal with the news.

I was very aware of wanting it to be a learning experience for those interns. I mentioned that I had called for a nurse quite a while ago for some pain medication, but no one had come. One of the interns interrupted and asked if I would like him to get the nurse. When he re-

---

[8] The gluteus maximus is the largest of the three gluteal muscles and makes up a large portion of the shape of the buttocks.

turned, I took his arm and told him he was going to be a wonderful doctor.

I asked Abby at what point her defenses lowered and the reality of her situation began to sink in at gut level. She said she did not think that had happened. Her style was to revert to an analytical, intellectual view of things. Throughout the process, she has been interested in noting her experience and discussing it with certain people in terms of what it means to be dying and how it affects her.

That being said, while the analytical approach is the primary psychological defense for me, there are different levels of understanding. So I wouldn't say that the analytical approach has dropped away, at least not yet. I'd say as different things have happened to me, whether it has been the start of chemo, or pain getting much worse, or levels of fatigue that demolish my defenses, I get jolted into a *Fuck me, this is for real* state. It's as if there is a firewall that keeps me safe from the consciousness of it, but there are moments when that firewall becomes very porous and the awareness of the fact that I am dying seeps in.

Sometimes when I experience something I really love, I suddenly realize I'm losing this, and it moves me closer to the reality of what is actually happening to me. I want to be present to what is happening. I've never experienced the mind/body connection as profoundly as I have recently. What ongoing, intense pain can do; what deep-down fatigue can do—we need a new word in our vocabulary because nothing that exists can describe it. At this point, most of the pain is under control with a great deal of medication.

The "how long do I have?" dance is a delicate one. I watch the oncologists move between realism and hope. It goes on all the time because no one can answer; no one can ever know.

Abby described her nineteen-year-old son as gentle and supportive. She has concerns about what he is actually feeling, since he is not particularly forthcoming. Her fifteen-year-old daughter is much more open about her feelings, but fifteen is a difficult age under any circumstances. They are able to sit around and laugh, cry, and talk in a way that Abby hopes is healing for her girl.

The most important thing for my kids is that they have already seen me defy expectations. I never took a medical leave from work and only recently was promoted to full professor. They have seen me move from a wheelchair to a walker, to a cane to my own legs, walking unassisted. My husband's view is interesting. He says that I still look pretty good, so no problem.

Early on after the diagnosis, I started thinking that I would probably live about two years. Of course, that was based on nothing. I could have lived two days or I might live another twenty years. Since then, I think I have become more hopeful partially because of a letter I wrote to the *New York Times*. It was about statistics and how they are out of date by the time they get into print. Besides, I'm not a statistic.

The assumption is we all want to live as long as pos-

sible, but if you saw me on one of those really bad days,
I might tell you that I don't want to go on living this way.
It's all about the quality of life. That remains to be seen.

ALLAN: **If you knew you had three months to live, is there
anything you would do differently?**
ABBY: No, absolutely not. I'm doing exactly what I want to do.
I'm also terribly aware of how fortunate I am. I have health insurance, I know how to speak with a doctor, I know what is going
on. Within my pain and misfortune, I am incredibly fortunate.

Jeff and Abby both live with a terminal diagnosis and each deals
with it quite differently. One has developed a whole new vision
of himself and the world and is living as the person he wants to
be. The other rejoices in the fact that she is doing exactly what
she wants with her remaining time. She too is living the life she
loves. The important thing is that they both spend their days
living, not dying. Each has healed in their own way.

To be born is to enter into a terminal condition. With compassion and wisdom as our guides, we can live every day fulfilling our vision. We can live our days honorably, with dignity, and
with grace.

GRATITUDE

A life without gratitude is a life asleep.
A life in which we cannot forgive is a life imprisoned.

On a recent Sunday morning I asked the people at the Community Meditation Center to consider the case of a man
who had been in a serious accident—a plane crash. He was

badly injured and the doctors said he would not survive his injuries. He incurred burns over one-third of his body, many of which were classified as "full thickness" (third-degree). He went through numerous surgeries, grafts, and other procedures. He had to relearn how to walk, and the use of his hands, while improving, is still limited. He did survive his injuries and is dealing well with the associated pain and inconveniences. He is now enjoying life with his family and is deeply involved in the work he finds most gratifying.

The question I asked folks to consider was whether they saw this man as fortunate or unfortunate. Most, knowing full well who the man was, felt that he was both unfortunate and fortunate. I, being the person most intimately familiar with this man, said that at this point the man saw himself as remarkably fortunate. It would be foolish to say that in the days immediately following his accident he thought about how fortunate he was. That would be unrealistic for one dealing with intense pain, confusion, and turmoil. But as the days and weeks passed, he began to see himself as truly blessed. Each day his heart became more and more filled with gratitude.

To frequently see oneself as unfortunate or unlucky is to plant the seed of victim mentality within one's own mind. No one gets everything they want, in the proportion they want, when they want it, all the time. To expect otherwise is to live in a state of delusion, and that too makes one into a victim—a "sad sack, poor me" unhappy being. Rarely, if ever, does one rejoice in life's most difficult moments, but when balanced with a true expression of gratitude for life's joyous times, and even simply for life itself, a brighter, more radiant existence unfolds.

On a more technical level, the work of Dr. Richard Davidson at the University of Wisconsin–Madison has been instrumental in showing that dharma/meditative practice alleviates negative (destructive) emotions. It does so by significantly altering the way in which the brain functions. Dr. Davidson has found that when people are caught up in strong, disturbing feelings such as fear, anger, and deep sadness, there is a great deal of activity in the amygdala, a structure in the emotional center of the brain. There is also a noticeably high level of activity in the right prefrontal cortex, located just behind the forehead.

The amygdala drives this part of the prefrontal cortex when we are caught up in negative emotions. When these emotions dominate, our thinking, perceptions, and memories are distorted and can have a streaming effect. Fear breeds more fear, anger, more anger, or as stated previously, whatever one reflects upon frequently becomes the inclination of the mind. We can become more and more negative about what we do not have and what is wrong, or more and more grateful for what we do have and for all that is right. It seems that we have a choice and that the practice of meditation can bring about a significant positive change.

It is extremely difficult to feel grateful when we are fearful or anxious. An illness, injury, or loss can certainly bring on anxiety, as can a disagreement with a loved one, or a tense business meeting. Starting with not feeling at our best, we wonder when and if we will ever feel at ease again. It can be difficult to remember that healing and serenity can only be experienced in the present moment. This is yet another instance where a contemplative practice such as meditation can be so beneficial.

Perhaps the most basic fear is that of not feeling safe. Safety is primary to our sense of well-being. Therefore, when we sense danger or a loss of security, fear can arise quickly. When I was caught in that plane and could not get out of the flames, I cried out for help, but it was immediately evident that no earthly help was coming. It was pure survival instinct that gave me the strength to tear myself free and jump from the plane. I sometimes think about how grateful I am that such a compulsion is part of the human mind/body nexus. I would most likely not be alive if it were otherwise.

It would be misleading to suggest that the practices offered herein will guarantee a safe and secure feeling all the time. In meditation, as an example, thoughts and emotions often arise accompanied by discomfort. That is why it is important to remember that nothing can come up that is not already within. The dark, unexplored corners of our mind yearn to heal and can only do so when light is shone upon them. We can accept in advance that such exploration might not always feel good, but at the same time we can be grateful for our own courage and fortitude.

An accident or serious illness often brings with it a sense of helplessness, a feeling that we have no control over the events in our life. Being laid off from our job or having our loved one leave us can bring up similar feelings. While it is not true that we have no control, it can be a highly disruptive realization to learn how little control we actually have. As we relinquish the delusion of believing that we are in control, we are actually offering ourselves a great gift, one for which we can be extremely grateful. Rather than creating a life of struggle in which we are constantly battling, we learn to ride the currents, skillfully discerning what we can change from what we cannot. We must also understand and accept that even when we choose to take action we may not be able to bring about the changes we want. That is why our motivation and full effort are of utmost importance for our peace of mind.

Under affliction in the very depths,
stop and contemplate what you have to be grateful for.
—MARY BAKER EDDY, *founder of Christian Science*

When bedridden or otherwise hampered by illness or injury, we may experience an identity crisis. When we are unable to carry on with our usual activities, it is not uncommon to feel a loss of purpose. We must face issues like an identity crisis or a sense of purposelessness realistically, because successfully traversing the healing journey requires that we proceed with the lightness of a bright heart. Loss, real or imagined, can weigh heavily upon us. Our daily activities—work, family, socializing, and the like—are important to us. They take up most of our waking hours. Yet there are times when we cannot be physically active. If we find that we cannot *do*, we must learn how to *be*.

Daily life presents us with ample opportunities to practice gratitude, most of which we tend to view as annoyances: waiting in line in the supermarket, traffic jams, airport delays, and so forth. From an idealistic point of view we can posture and say that we should not have to practice gratitude. We should simply be grateful. On a spiritually lofty level that may be true, but in a real-world, earthly existence it may not always be so. The ubiquitous nature of dukkha requires of us a conscious approach to gratitude if we are to avoid the bleakness of loneliness and despair.

People are not grateful because they are happy,
They are happy because they are grateful.
—BR. DAVID STEINDL-RAST

Gratitude is one of the fastest-acting remedies available to us. One moment, one quick reminder to ourselves of all that we have to be grateful for will lift our spirits. Meditation, on the other hand, while of extraordinary value, takes time to develop, as does physical fitness. Gratitude is instantaneous. When we look deeply, no matter what has befallen us, there is always something for which to be grateful. My friend, the great Native American sculptor Michael Naranjo, was blinded and lost the use of most of his right hand in the Vietnam War. He told me that although there were times when he was frightened, he always knew that he would be all right because he was alive and his mind was clear. For that, he was grateful.

When we hear about a friend who has been diagnosed with cancer, or another who has been injured in an accident, or a neighbor whose husband has died, we might think, *How can I complain about my fractured ankle? I should be grateful.* But suffering and distress are not comparative matters. There is no prize for the person who suffers the most. We can have great compassion for those who are under duress, but that embraces all beings, including ourselves. No one goes through life without experiencing dukkha. Gratitude is a practice that can dramatically change the way we deal with misfortune. Illness, old age, accidents, and abusiveness can all push gratefulness out of our hearts.

Our practice is to be present to all that is, not just fragments of the whole. We are not just elderly, or ill, or one who has been injured. There is much more to all of us, and in the whole being there is much for which each of us can be grateful. As author Agatha Christie said, "I have sometimes been wildly, despairingly, acutely miserable . . . but through it all I still know quite certainly that just to be alive is a grand thing."

I HAVE a friend who keeps a gratitude journal. At the end of each day she writes down five things that she has experienced during that day for which she feels grateful. She loves keeping the journal and feels that it grounds her. I can certainly see value in the practice, although I myself am more of an "in the moment" kind of guy. I allow myself to bask in the feelings that come up when I hold my wife in my arms (has it really been twenty-two years?); when the final moments of the Mahler Second Symphony wash over and transport me to the heavens; when that adorable five-year-old imp shrieks, "Hi, Grandpa"; when his mom cannot contain her joy because she just closed a big deal; when the little green shoots peek out after winter's long dark night; when the neighbor's chocolate Labrador licks my nose; and when my sangha laughs at one of my silly jokes.

Death almost had me, and one day it surely will. For now, however, I am grateful for each day of life.

KARMA

Karma is a Sanskrit word that translates as "action." However, because Buddhist teachings place such significance on our actions, the single word "action" is not sufficient to adequately express the profound nature of karma. In fact, the Buddha said that only a fully awakened being could comprehend the complete and far-reaching meaning of karma. A dictionary definition would likely speak of the law of causality, or conditionality, in which the intentions and deeds of an individual influence their future. In the Western world, that has evolved into the rather simplified view that good deeds produce good karma, while bad deeds produce bad karma—a type of "what goes around comes around" concept. The Buddha understood that we often have little control over the results of our actions. He therefore taught that our karmic imprint is determined not by the results of our actions but by the intention that motivates those actions.

A popular misconception related to karma is that it is a form of fate or destiny, and therefore we are incapable of changing it. Further, the connotation is that karma is usually negative. "It's my bad karma. It always rains on my birthday." Only limited harm will come from such foolish thinking. When it can get serious is if we start having thoughts like, *I was in that accident because of my bad karma*, or *His cancer is because of his negative karma*. The danger in this type of thinking is its potential to undermine compassion. If we think that we are suffering because of our karma, we can easily believe that we are not worthy of self-compassion or kindness from others, or that others, in turn, are not worthy of our compassion.

The Buddhist view of karma is more expansive and nonlinear. I was injured in an accident because of the way conditions came together in a specific moment. That moment was preceded by, and influenced by, what came before it, including my past actions. But I do not believe that I was being punished for some awful deed I might have committed in the past. This view, based on the law of cause and effect, is grounded in logic, not retribution. It also helps us to see that we are not helpless victims of past actions. (Some Buddhist scholars might say that we have been reborn so many times—from before beginningless time—that we have committed every conceivable action. Therefore, there would be a karmic relation between my previous actions and that plane crash. On such matters I am fairly agnostic.)

If the weather report tells us that driving our car during current icy conditions is dangerous, we can make the decision not to drive to the market until those conditions change. If the doctor advises us that losing a few pounds would help us avoid heart problems, we can make the decision to pay more attention to our diet and exercise. From this perspective, we see that karma is multifaceted and that what happens in this moment is influenced by both past and present deeds. Our actions in this moment are influenced by the past and we are creating our experience of the present. At the same time, we are also shaping our experience of the future.

So while our decisions in the present are somewhat influenced by our past actions, we still have free will. We get to make choices. That brings us back to living mindfully. Our parents, our upbringing, and the various influences in our life are significant, but not nearly as important as our motivations that determine our current actions. The various inequities that we have experienced in the past are part of who we are, but it is what we do right now that matters most.

When we are certain of the motivations that generate our current actions, we will have insight and understanding of the term "karma," and we will be living in the present.

HUMOR

Never lose your sense of humor" is a lovely thought and often offered at seminars and workshops. I have a good sense of humor. I love to laugh and help others laugh. A few years ago, I would have thought it possible to always keep my sense of humor active no matter what the situation. Now I know that is not true. For several months, my life felt so bleak that I do not remember any laughter other than perhaps at an occasional ironic situation.

There are times when the realities of life present us with a severe loss. Such a loss can be felt in every cell and every fiber of our existence. Our sense of humor abandons us for a while and we grieve as we must. Somehow, the extraordinary resilience of the human being perseveres, and we go on. Our sense of humor returns and is ready to lighten our load.

I was aware that my laughter was absent, and I sorely missed it. Fortunately, it is hard to keep a good sense of humor down. It giggles beneath the surface, tickles your innards, and cries out to be released and bring joy to you and those around you. I wanted this so much that I looked for any opportunity to bring humor back into my life. Now, here I am with pains and scars, but as jovial as ever. A sense of humor has brought lightness to my healing process.

What do you call a dinosaur with an extensive vocabulary?
A thesaurus.

Through the centuries, a great deal of research has been done probing for the curative properties of humor. The term "humor" comes from the humoral medicine of the ancient Greeks, who believed that the balance of fluids in the human body, known as "humours," controlled human health and emotions. Modern-day research has served to reiterate what most of us already knew: Laughter has a sense of relaxation about it, therefore, a corresponding feeling of less stress.

Laughing out loud, or even a gentle smile, can neutralize negative feelings temporarily. While that may not seem like much, it can be the beginning of coming out of hell. One thing we know for sure, laughter feels good, and there are times when even a moment of good feeling can feel *really* good. It may not provide a cure but it can sure help us heal.

> *There's a new restaurant in town called Karma.*
> *There's no menu; they just give you what you deserve.*

JOY

After a while, my examinations at the hospital were scaled back to a visit every three months. On one of those occasions as Dr. Yurt was examining my hands, I felt a wave of envy surge through me with such intensity that it caused me to shiver. His hands—his talented, highly skilled surgeon's hands—were perfect. They were strong, with straight fingers and neatly manicured nails. My hands were scarred, weak, and tremulous. My fingers were twisted, and all of my fingernails were gone, melted away by fire. The sadness I felt was deep; all perspective was lost.

Then, as quickly as those feelings had arisen, they faded away. I thought to myself, *Dr. Yurt's hands are of great benefit to many. They relieve pain and sorrow. My hands are healing. They will never again look the way they did, but each day they are getting stronger and more capable. How wonderful that people benefit from Dr. Yurt's hands. How amazing that function is returning to mine.*

THERE IS a teaching that in Sanskrit is called *mudita*. It means "sympathetic joy," or my own favorite translation, "harmonious joy." However translated, mudita is about experiencing joy at the good fortune and happiness of another. It is a quality that encourages us to relate to the success and happiness of others with delight. It frees us from envy and greed. Mudita is particularly challenging if we feel the other did not deserve their good fortune, or if we believe it came at our expense.

(Mudita has no one-word translation in English but, interestingly enough, its opposite does. "Schadenfreude" means taking joy, delight, or pleasure at the misfortune of another.)

Craving brings us unhappiness in the forms of jealousy, envy, and greed. Mudita diminishes that unhappiness, as well as that of enmity, ill will, and impatience. A Spanish proverb says, "The door to the human heart can be opened only from the inside." Mudita opens the door to kindness and compassion. Mudita, however, can also bring us face-to-face with some interesting questions: Do we feel intimidated by the success of others? Do we believe that the success or happiness of another can diminish our own? Do we evaluate our selves based on comparisons with others? Do we fear another person's success can take from ours?

The practice of mudita begins with taking note of our emotional state when we resent someone else's good fortune. What kind of environment are we creating in our own minds? Examine your inner landscape. Experiencing harmonious joy will be challenging at times. It is easier to practice mudita if you are doing well and the other person's good fortune does not feel like a threat. But if you are not doing as well as you would like and the other person gets what you want, it is more difficult to feel happy for her. It can help to remember that the amount of happiness available to all of us is not limited. No one else can use up yours.

I HAVE personal and painful experience with the dangers of fire. In his teachings, the Buddha often uses "fire" metaphorically to describe powerful internal dangers. He speaks of the fire of craving for possessions and more and more pleasures; the fire of begrudging the success of others; the fire of envy that comes when others gain; the fire of comparing ourselves with someone we see as having greater status than we have. Mudita cools these fires.

Feel free to experiment. Start by becoming more aware of something good that has happened to someone you like. Take a moment to be with their happiness. Move on to someone you do not even know, perhaps someone you read about or heard about on television. Take a moment to feel her joy. Ultimately, you may even be able to share the happiness of someone you do not even like. It is not easy if they can walk and you cannot, or if they can see and you are sightless. They may be wealthy while you are struggling. They may be dating the person you think is hot.

What would it feel like to allow in the joy of someone else's good fortune? When we can view the happiness of others with joy and equanimity, then we are diminishing our own greed and craving. We are increasing our own happiness. We are in the process of ending suffering.

EQUANIMITY

The dictionary defines equanimity as "mental calmness, composure, and evenness of temper, especially in difficult situations." In Sanskrit, the word that translates as equanimity is *upekkha*, which means, "to look over" (not "overlook," which is entirely different). It refers to the evenness of mind that arises from straightforward observation and insight. It is the calm that exists when we see into the nature of phenomena without being caught up in what we see. We know only the bare experience without the subjective add-ons that we create.

Thus equanimity, when well developed, can lead to a sense of ease and inner peace, even in times of disruption. Whether the moment is pleasant or unpleasant, the mind remains composed. Equanimity is an invaluable quality throughout life, but especially when we are not at our best, as is usually the case when we are dealing with adversity. Equanimity is an invaluable practice that is its own reward—a sense of peace.

Another quality of equanimity is that it helps us to see the bigger picture. A feeling of spaciousness arises around a particular situation so that our view is not restricted. So equanimity sometimes evokes the connotation "to see with patience" or "to see with understanding." As an example, when we do not take the words of another personally, we are less likely to react aggressively to those words. There is then a greater possibility that we will respond with wisdom and compassion.

Equanimity is characterized by an active, alert state of mind. It is not apathy, indifference, or boredom. Effort and determination are required to develop equanimity. It is not just a feeling that blows in and wafts away of its own accord like an evening breeze. It is worth the effort to refine because when equanimity is present, suffering is minimized.

We can penetrate even deeper into the quality of equanimity by examining the Pali word *tatramajjhattata*, a compound made of three words. *Tatra* means "there," *majjha* means "middle," and *tata* means "to stand." Together, the word becomes "to stand there in the middle." This "standing in the middle" refers to maintaining a sense of balance while in the midst of whatever is happening. This kind of composure comes from inner strength, mindfulness, and integrity, all admirable qualities in their own right.

A prerequisite for the development of equanimity is acceptance. Equanimity helps us to see more clearly what is acceptable and what is not, and helps us maintain that clarity when deciding if and how to act. Equanimity arises from compassion and love. The Buddha described an equanimous mind as "abundant, exalted, immeasurable, and without hostility or ill will."

Equanimity allows us to be present to all situations, understanding that everything is as it has to be. That does not mean that everything is as we would like it to be, or that everything is pleasant or fair. It means that all circumstances are born of the causes and conditions that precede and accompany them. To change what is unpleasant, unjust, unkind, or unfair, we must change the causes and conditions. Our past actions have brought us to this moment. Our actions *in* this moment create our future, both for the rest of this day and for all our tomorrows.

As WE look at life, we see how the worldly winds blow, with the potential to toss us from pleasure to pain, gain to loss, praise to blame, and fame to obscurity. We are hoisted up and then discarded, we are healthy and then ill, we are waltzing and we twist an ankle. Rise and fall, delight and despair; do not get too comfortable because it will change, but then again do not get too concerned because it will change again. In this tangle of emotions called life, we find the courage to start anew as often as is necessary. We develop the insight that finds peace even as we deal with illness, calm even within a broken body. We balance compassion with wisdom to develop an unshakable stability of mind—we breathe in the dignity of equanimity.

Equanimity is grounded in active awareness (insight). It is not indifference, laziness, or dullness of mind. It is earned through diligent training and is not to be confused with a passing mood. At the same time, there is an ease about equanimity that allows it to be present without strenuous effort being expended again and again. Equanimity strengthens itself but only if it has been developed and sustained by insight.

We want to have an equanimous view of all beings, including those whom we do not even like. When it comes to our loved ones, it can be difficult to develop a mind of nonattachment, yet it is possible and indeed imperative to do so if we are to alleviate stress. It is understood that we might experience a certain degree of attachment in our closest relationships, but attachment and possessiveness are the basic ingredients of suffering. It is not easy to be in a meaningful and loving relationship without forming attachments, but we can love without being possessive. We can feel pleasure without becoming addicted or greedy. We can feel angry without seeking revenge. To do so requires that we live fully present to the joys and sorrows of each moment.

I definitely lost the peace of equanimity in my first days home from the hospital. I wanted things to be the way they used to be. I did not want so much pain and loss. That was perfectly understandable, but it was also the exact formula for suffering. Clinging to a desire for things to be different than they are spells dukkha. Fortunately, it did not take too long for me to remember that life comprises both joys and sorrows. This was my time to experience an extremely difficult situation, but I did not have to suffer. I reminded myself again and again of the impermanent nature of all things, or as it is sometimes said, "This too shall pass." The more I accepted, the more I again enjoyed the peace of an equanimous mind.

The extent of my injuries have made for a formidable teacher. But my injuries and I are not at war. We are partners forging a new path—one in which we are learning to function effectively and joyfully.

DEATH

Defying medical opinion, I did not die on Christmas Day 2012, but approximately 168,000 others did. That is about how many people around the world die each day. It is a daily occurrence, the most natural, commonplace, ordinary, and reliable of all phenomena. The most basic of all laws of the universe is—that which is born will die. It is the true nature of all things. The only way to avoid death is to not be born, and for me, it is a little late for that.

Your death may be deeply felt by a small number of people, but no matter who dies, the world goes on. Death is an everyday occurrence. It is not a calamity, or repulsive, or despicable, and it is certainly not optional. It is ordinary, and at the same time it is truly a once-in-a-lifetime occurrence. We all know we are going to die, but do we really accept it at our deepest gut level? Is there a little cellular piece of you hidden away in a corner of your mind that believes you will be the first exception?

The obituary column tells us who has died, while across the page the birth announcements introduce the newcomers. If death and after-death questions cause anxiety and concern, and you absolutely must have answers, religions can provide them for you. The problem, of course, is that even as the preacher is extolling the virtues of heaven and eternal life, a part of us might be wondering, *How does he know?*

We live in a society conditioned to ignore death, which may

be why at the time of dying, many feel unprepared, confused, and frightened. Fortunately, we are showing signs of progress. Palliative care is rapidly growing in acceptance and sophistication. Hospice care is expanding exponentially. The World Health Organization describes palliative care as "an approach that improves the quality of life of patients and their families facing the problems associated with life-threatening illness, through the prevention and relief of suffering by means of the early identification and impeccable assessment and treatment of pain and other problems, physical, psychosocial and spiritual."

Over the past twenty-five years, the focus on a patient's quality of death has greatly increased. It is estimated that more than 55 percent of larger hospitals (those with a hundred or more beds) in the United States offer some sort of palliative care program. These efforts must be supported since they can bring comfort at a time of life that may otherwise be disconcerting and frightening.

Even though we have experienced the death of friends and relatives and we know that everything is short-lived, so many of us ignore preparing for our own death. That ignorance fertilizes fear. We see others dying all the time, but we continue with our plan to file for an exception, or at least an extension. In the Hindu epic "Mahabharata," the learned Yudhisthira is asked, "Of all things in life, what is the most amazing?" His reply, "That a man, although seeing others die all around him, still thinks he will not die."

I read about a woman who, reflecting on when her cancer had been diagnosed as terminal, said, "Being terminal just meant that at last I acknowledged that death was real. It did not mean that I would die in six weeks or six months or even die before the doctor who had given me my prognosis. It simply meant that I acknowledged that I would die."

To have a good death, we must lead a good life: compassionate, loving, generous, joyful, and wise. We must make the decisions that create such a life. For a good death, the Buddha said, "Prepare now." "Impermanent are all conditioned things," he taught. "Strive on with diligence." It is wise to live every moment of our lives as the person we want to be. We know that person. No matter what the current state of our body, that person lives within us, ready to join in the healing process, no matter what still remains to be remedied.

There is no need to fear the true nature of life, which in turn can help us prepare for our death. Such preparation need not feel morbid. In fact, it can lead to a true sense of liberation. Try reflecting regularly on these five subjects for contemplation:[9]

I am of the nature to grow old; I cannot avoid aging.
I am of the nature to be ill; I cannot avoid illness.
I am of the nature to die; I cannot avoid death.
All that is dear to me, and everyone I love, are of the nature to change.
I will be separated from all that is dear and loved by me.
I am the owner of my actions. My actions are my only true belongings. My actions are the ground on which I stand.

For most of us, our fear of dying is a fear of the unknown. The two operative words being "fear" and "unknown." When it

---

[9] The Buddha, *Upajjhatthana Sutta, Anguttara Nikaya* 5.7.

comes to death, there is not much that we can do about the "unknown" part. We do not get to check out death, determine that it is safe, and then come back reassured to finish our natural life. Therefore, all we can work with is the "fear" part. Fortunately, we understand that fear is a feeling. When it comes to the subject of death, the feeling can be quite intense. But no matter how compelling it is, fear remains just a feeling. As discussed earlier, fear is about something that we believe might happen in the future. There is no "might" when it comes to death. It *will* happen in the future. How far into the future is unknown. Our concerns would seem to be about what the experience itself will be like and what actually happens after this life has ended.

Even though I came close to death, I can offer no insights into what death itself is like. There seems to be only one way to find out, and those who have found out do not report back. (There are those who would disagree and say that they have come back from the dead, but I have a pretty strong skeptical streak within me. I also remain agnostic on the subject of rebirth.)

I believe it would be a great gift to ourselves to be fully present to our own death. The termination of a life cycle is surely as significant, if not more so, than its dawning. There would be so much to learn. Yet the reality remains that we cannot know about death without dying.

When I first became seriously interested in the process of dying, I made up a meditative practice that did a great deal to alleviate my fears. I envisioned myself lying on a bed and approaching my death. When I first tried, it was emotionally quite unnerving, but the better I became at the practice, the closer I could envision myself at the edge of death. At first, the closer I got to the edge the more frightening the experience. Then the fear began to dissipate and I was left with just the experience. Of course, I could take myself only to the edge of death because without the actual experience of dying, that was as far as I could go.

I did not tell many people about this practice because I thought that I might be viewed as somewhat wacky. Later on, as I did gradually begin to share my experience, I found people to be quite interested, especially when I told them that through this exercise my fear of dying had been greatly diminished. Fear is a major form of suffering, and practices that alleviate fear should be investigated. If you try this practice, go slowly and take the time to observe your feelings. One thing that all my years in the theater taught me was that good hard work in rehearsal made the actual performance easier and better.

I also learned a great deal from Sogyal Rinpoche's extraordinary *The Tibetan Book of Living and Dying*. I am not Tibetan and not every concept in the book was right for me, but the in-depth description of the dying process itself helped me feel more prepared for death than I had ever been. To state the obvious, fear of the unknown is reduced when one knows more.

When our role is that of caretaker to a dying person, we can experience overwhelming and deeply moving feelings as we sit with them. We may bear witness to grieving relatives or come face-to-face with our own sadness, confusion, and fear. Practices such as meditation, compassion, patience, generosity, and forgiveness help us develop insight and alleviate stress and angst. We gain greater resiliency and stability.

Skills that we use in formal meditation practice can also be applied to short periods of contemplation, so that we can regain our equanimity while dealing with stressful situations. Observing the in-breath and out-breath for just one minute can restore inner peace. The Vietnamese monk Thich Nhat Hanh used to teach us a simple way to regain tranquility. Stop everything and bring your awareness to the next breath and say to yourself, *Breathing in, I am calm. Breathing out, I smile.* In truth you may not feel at all calm, but there is something persuasive about this "power of positive breathing."

Silence can feel awkward, but often it is the most noble of gifts. When my brother was dying, I sometimes sat with him for long periods of time with neither of us speaking. One time he said to me, "Are you comfortable with all this silence?" I replied, "Yes, how about you?" "Yes, me too." Then after a pause he added, "The others talk too much."

Michael was a caretaker to his wife, Faith, from the time she was diagnosed with posterior cortical atrophy in 2002 until her death in 2008.[10] "I started noticing her lack of focus and that her spatial skills were off. She would actually hit the wall of the garage when pulling the car in. I developed tremendous fear and would sometimes become irritated with her because of my fear. It was confusing and disruptive."

The doctors said they knew little about the disease and there was nothing they could do to treat her. Michael felt a sense of hopelessness and despair. He had to deal with the reality that she was going to die and there was nothing he could do about it. She never lost a sense of herself, as happens with Alzheimer's. She remained fully aware of what was happening to her, which Michael described as "devastating to watch." He became her sole caretaker.

---

[10] Posterior cortical atrophy (PCA) is a form of dementia that is usually considered an atypical variant of Alzheimer's disease.

The long progression downward continued. Michael began drinking, and during the course of Faith's illness he gained seventy pounds. At night he would feed her and get her ready for bed. Then he would be alone with his feelings and they would be overwhelming. "I had never felt anything like it. I didn't know that level of despair existed, and I didn't know that level of love existed."

He became so worn out that the doctor told him he would not outlive her. He finally agreed to bring in help. He was wiped out. He had nothing left. There was nothing more for him to do except to love her, cherish her, and keep her safe until she died.

Advances in modern medicine and technology over the past twenty to thirty years have done a great deal to alleviate one of the main fears of many people—that of experiencing extreme suffering in the days leading up to their death. Today there are medications that can significantly ease pain while the patient remains quite lucid. In many instances the patient can actually control the amount of medication being administered.

Research shows that most people would prefer not to die in a hospital, yet that is exactly where some 55 percent of Americans die. While it is not always possible to have everything as we would like, it is still advisable to make your wishes known in writing. An "advance health care directive" is one type of document used for that purpose. (See discussion in the Appendix on various alternatives.)

When to die—the moral and legal aspects of euthanasia—is a highly charged issue that, if being considered, must be thoroughly examined and understood. A great deal of research is available for patients, family members, and medical professionals.

The American Civil Liberties Union stated in its 1996 amicus[11] brief in *Vacco* v. *Quill* that:

> The right of a competent, terminally ill person to avoid excruciating pain and embrace a timely and dignified death bears the sanction of history and is implicit in the concept of ordered liberty. The exercise of this right is as central to personal autonomy and bodily integrity as rights safeguarded by this Court's decisions relating to marriage, family relationships, procreation, contraception, child rearing, and the refusal or termination of life-saving medical treatment. In particular, this Court's recent decisions concerning the right to refuse medical treatment and the right to abortion instruct that a mentally competent, terminally ill person has a protected liberty interest in choosing to end intolerable suffering by bringing about his or her own death.
>
> A state's categorical ban on physician assistance to suicide—as applied to competent, terminally ill patients who wish to avoid unendurable pain and hasten inevitable death—substantially interferes with this protected liberty interest and cannot be sustained.

The American Medical Association (AMA) stated in a June 1994 report "Decisions near the End of Life":

---

[11] In legal terms, "amicus" refers to an impartial advisor, often voluntary, to a court of law in a specific case.

It is understandable, though tragic, that some patients in extreme duress—such as those suffering from a terminal, painful, debilitating illness—may come to decide that death is preferable to life. However, permitting physicians to engage in euthanasia would ultimately cause more harm than good. Euthanasia is fundamentally incompatible with the physician's role as healer, would be difficult or impossible to control, and would pose serious societal risks.

The involvement of physicians in euthanasia heightens the significance of its ethical prohibition. The physician who performs euthanasia assumes unique responsibility for the act of ending the patient's life. Euthanasia could also readily be extended to incompetent patients and other vulnerable populations.

Instead of engaging in euthanasia, physicians must aggressively respond to the needs of patients at the end of life. Patients should not be abandoned once it is determined that cure is impossible. Patients near the end of life must continue to receive emotional support, comfort care, adequate pain control, respect for patient autonomy, and good communication.

Buddhist teachings view euthanasia, or assisted suicide, as an error in judgment, since it is in violation of the most basic Buddhist belief to abstain from the destruction of life. The counterargument is the Buddhist emphasis on the development and practice of compassion and the alleviation of suffering. The Dalai Lama has suggested that all situations of this type be evaluated on an individual case-by-case basis.

Many Christians believe that taking a life, for any reason, is interfering with God's plan and is essentially murder. Conservative Christians are usually against even passive euthanasia.[12] Some Christians take the other side of the argument and believe that the drugs to end suffering early are God-given and should be used when there is no known possibility of recovery.

Judaism believes that only God has the right to extinguish life. The body is essentially the property of God, and no one has the right to decide the fate of a living body. Judaism teaches that life, no less than death, is involuntary. Only the Creator, who bestows the gift of life, may take away that life, even when it has become a burden rather than a blessing.

Muslims are opposed to euthanasia. They believe that all human life is sacred. Life is given only by Allah, and only Allah chooses how long each person will live. Human beings should not interfere in this. Many devout Muslims believe that Do Not Resuscitate (DNR) orders represent a soft form of euthanasia and therefore are in opposition to Islamic law.

COMPASSIONATE AND skillful action would seem less about strictly following dogmatic teachings or precepts than about the specifics of a given situation. It would mean that patient, caretaker, and medical staff would pay close attention to the dying person and take the time necessary to evaluate what would be in the best interest of the patient. This would indeed be a formidable task and a great honor, one that could move each

---

[12] Passive euthanasia is the hastening of the death of a person by altering some form of support and letting nature take its course. Examples include such things as turning off respirators, halting medications, and discontinuing food and water so as to allow a person to dehydrate or starve to death.

human being toward a more comfortable and less confusing end of life.

WISDOM

Wijsheid; Weisheit; Saggezza; Sabiduria; Visdom;
Hekima; Sagesse; Eagna; Doethineb[13]

Wisdom is a quality that has been revered in every culture in the civilized world throughout the ages. It is an attribute earned, and not easily so. As Confucius said, "By three ways do we acquire wisdom: the first is by contemplation, which is the noblest; the second is by imitation, which is the easiest; the third is by experience, which is the bitterest." Wisdom is developed through wise thinking and wise actions. Knowledge, intellect, and success are not wisdom, although they can be contributing factors. Only personal experience leads to wisdom.

Knowledge is knowing that a tomato is a fruit.
Wisdom is not putting one in a fruit salad.

The Buddha had a way to measure wisdom: You are wise to the extent that you can get yourself to do things you do not like because you can see that they will lead to happiness, and to not do things you like because you see that they will lead to unhappiness. Wisdom has to outwit narrow-minded preferences in order to yield sustainable happiness.

---

[13] The word "wisdom" in Dutch, German, Italian, Spanish, Norwegian, Swahili, French, Irish, and Welsh.

Wisdom arises from integrity, which requires a sincere interest in examining our intentions. When we have acted unskillfully, we must be willing to own up so that we do not repeat actions that harm ourselves or others. Confronting the truth in this way may not always feel very good. It is the brambly, stony part of the path that leads to awakening.

Knowing yourself is the beginning of all wisdom.
—ARISTOTLE

The person who listens with an open mind, carefully examines details, and takes their time before coming to conclusions, rather than simply accepting the first opinion that is offered, is more likely to develop wisdom. The path of just accepting popular belief is easy. The path of awakening requires patience, courage, and intelligence. The truth of Aristotle's words has not altered through the ages: "Knowing yourself is the beginning of all wisdom."

The development of wisdom requires living truthfully and peacefully, with kindness, compassion, and generosity. The essence of wisdom is to see through to the true nature of things. The expression "beginner's mind" suggests that we not be burdened by preconceptions but rather develop a spirited curiosity with room for insight and growth and a more perceptive use of knowledge.

It is wise to remember that suffering relates in some way to wanting things to be different from the way they are. Things *are* the way they are and often acceptance is the wisest action. Our view of a difficult situation is not fixed and solid. It can change. A useful practice is to stop, close your eyes, and consider how your stress and discomfort with a particular situation might be eased if you could accept things as they are, at least for now. It is often difficult to see, but every negative situation holds within it the potential for renewal and awakening.

THE WISEST among us can still experience anger and frustration, but they understand that those are feelings. They wait to speak or act until the heat of the moment has subsided. It is often wise to ask yourself if you are about to act as the person you want to be. Physical pain and the frustrations that can accompany an illness or loss can weaken our resolve and lead to words that we later regret. With insight, we are aware of what we are experiencing and can act more wisely. This means specifically refraining from acting or speaking while under the influence of disturbing emotions. It is hard to put your foot in your mouth when it is closed.

In Buddhist texts there is a great deal of emphasis on overcoming suffering. In the process we empathize with the suffering of others and cultivate compassion for all beings. There is little that is more beneficial for one's own healing than reaching out and focusing on the needs of others.

It is wisdom that enables us to see beyond ego and gain clarity where there might otherwise be confusion. If we cling to vengeful thoughts directed toward the person we feel has hurt us, or the doctor whose surgery did not fix all that we had hoped for, we will surely be derailing our train from the way to wisdom. That is not to say that people should not be held responsible for their actions, but we must pay careful attention to what goes on in our mind so that we act wisely. We can never know the whole story about anything.

An open, loving heart is a major factor in healing and finding happiness. When we are not burdened by clinging to anger, resentment, and bitterness, our journey becomes more manageable. Even when facing life's most challenging situations we can still be open to moments of peace and grace. Holding on to negative feelings hardens the heart and closes us off from the happiness that can be ours, even during difficult times. When we hold on to anger because of what we feel another person has done, or what the world has done to us, we are not being wise.

Bitterness can overtake us when we believe our difficult circumstance can never change. When we see that any situation can—and will—change, however, we are seeing things as they really are, and that is the ground of wisdom. It is also wise to do what we can to encourage the change within ourselves that will free us from resentment and bitterness. It is not situations and conditions that cause our happiness and unhappiness, but how we experience those situations.

Understanding that our thoughts, feelings, and sensations are not reality is essential to the development of wisdom. They may be incredibly intense, but they are still just thoughts, feelings, and sensations. Without understanding the difference we may find ourselves acting on any thought that happens to pass through our mind, and that is definitely not wise. This insight can help us think, speak, and act with greater clarity. When we do not see things clearly, we can easily become overwhelmed by fear.

It takes time to develop wisdom so we tend to associate it with our seniors. That is usually a safe bet, but of course we have all known some old fools and we have met some wise children. Wisdom does not always come with age. Sometimes age comes all by itself. All beings, knowledgeable or not, intelligent or not, experienced or not, have something to teach us. Listening is a skill honed by the wise.

Less than a year and a half after the plane crash, I heard something within me revealing what I never would have thought possible. If there were some sort of magic pill or supernatural power that could allow me to turn back the clock so that I would not have been in that accident, I would decline. I would choose to stay with my life as it is. I would not have said that a few months ago and I certainly would not have said it before the accident. But now, even with the pain, scarring, and struggles in my daily life, I would not go back.

Encountering death has taught me so much about life that I could never have learned any other way. I have seen what I could never have seen, felt what I could never have felt. I have experienced love and compassion on a level that I could never have imagined. Mostly, opportunities to serve my fellow beings have opened up that would not have happened otherwise.

I am in the latter part of my life, meaning that I have lived more days than I have left to live. To have these opportunities at this stage of my life is something too precious to give back. People seem to listen differently to someone who has beaten the odds; who has felt death's insidious fingers around his throat and been able to pry himself loose, at least temporarily. I want to use these days in the most meaningful ways possible. I have no idea what tomorrow will bring, but today is overflowing with potential.

One day in early November 2013, I went for my occupational therapy appointment in the hospital, and while I was waiting for the elevator, a woman walked up to me and said, "Paul." "No," I replied, "Allan." She said, "Oh, yes, Allan. Do you remember me?" I looked carefully. "No, I'm sorry." "I'm Mary," she said, "I was one of your nurses in the burn unit." "I'm afraid I was in bad shape at that time," I replied, "I don't think I would recognize anyone from the burn unit." "Oh, that's okay," she responded. "You look fantastic. I can't believe how good you look. We all thought you were . . . I mean . . . We thought you were going to . . ." I helped her out. "You thought I was going to die." "Well, your injuries were so bad. Your burns were"—a pause as she swallowed—"but you were always so kind . . . *so* kind." The elevator door opened and I said, "I'm afraid I have to go, I have a therapy appointment. It was good to see you." She stopped me and said, "May I give you a quick hug?" "Of course." As I held her I could feel her start to sob. She wiped her eyes and said, "I'm sorry, I'm just so happy you're okay." "Thank you," I replied. "Me too."

The elevator doors closed and the crowded car ascended slowly to the eighteenth floor. I thought once again about how, when someone suffers injuries to the extent that I had, they do not usually get to chat about it a year later. Gratitude, humility, and awe swept through every fiber of my being. I had survived. I was alive. Why and how barely hold passing interest anymore. What I do with my remaining time means everything. Above all else, when I am finished with my days, may those who knew me say, "He was so kind."

- You must practice a practice for it to be effective.
- Mindfulness is a wholesome, moment-to-moment, non-judgmental, engaged level of awareness.
- Patience requires wisdom, courage, and compassion.
- Live life as the person you want to be.
- There are many reasons not to be generous, but none of them brings happiness.
- It is a powerful practice to be generous when you are the one feeling in need.
- We can make the choices that lead to different results and greater happiness.
- Our life can be transformed by even a minimal change in our perceptions.
- The miraculous human body will verify the faith we have in it.
- Every negative situation holds within it the potential for renewal and awakening.
- It is often wise to ask yourself if you are about to act as the person you want to be.
- We create change by changing conditions, not by trying to change results.
- If we are too busy to be kind, we are too busy.
- No one is able to give to another the gift of happiness. Each of us has to cultivate it for ourselves.

- Any feelings of unhappiness exist within ourselves and therefore can only be changed within ourselves.
- You are not alone; everyone goes through difficult, even unbearable times.
- Surely there is no such thing as a stranger in this world.
- A moment of kindness, a compassionate smile, not only can uplift another being, it can save a life.
- Determination strengthens determination.
- Although victimized, we do not have to think of ourselves as a victim.
- Even a momentary pause can help you see things more clearly.
- Our entire quality of life can be impacted by minimal mental adjustments.
- Mindfulness is learned slowly, so allow yourself to experience the joys of small progress.
- Craving for tomorrow cheats us of today.
- The present is the only time we can experience all the joys, beauty, and delights life has to offer.
- When equanimity is present, suffering is not.
- People are not grateful because they are happy, they are happy because they are grateful.
- Do not allow yourself to be held captive by your thoughts and emotions.
- In reality there is no duality.
- To have a good death, we must lead a good life.
- The development of wisdom is the responsibility of each individual.
- A moment of gratitude is a sincere expression of an enlightened being.

- No one is more worthy of your love and tenderness than you are yourself.
- The world might not be perfect, but it is a good thing, a great and wondrous thing.
- Patience with self is essential if we are to enjoy happiness.
- Patience requires wisdom, courage, and compassion.
- The secret is not to seek love, but to offer love.
- It is more productive to focus on things as they are rather than what might have been.
- Live each day honorably, with dignity and with grace.
- A life in which we cannot forgive is a life imprisoned.
- Consider often what kind of environment you are creating in your mind.
- We have no idea what tomorrow will bring, but today is overflowing with potential.

ACKNOWLEDGMENTS

There is nothing like writing a book to demonstrate the nature of interconnectedness. Any sense of "I, me, or mine" melds into the reality of a collective "we" in which each component is indispensible. For *Through the Flames* the indispensables begin with the Tarcher/Penguin/Random House people who have offered their skills and enthusiasm for this, my third book with them; my editor and friend, Sara Carder, who is a creative joy to work with, as is her assistant, Joanna Ng; and the entire editorial team, led by publisher Joel Fotinos. Brianna Yamashita does a fantastic job leading the publicity folks as they let the world know that *Through the Flames* is hot. Thank you, Lauren Lucaire, for the magnificent eye-catching book jacket. Dorian Hastings lent invaluable advice and editorial support.

My special thanks to Sharon Salzberg, who has been such a supportive friend and guide through the years, and especially during my recovery period. Thank you, Sharon, for always being there with wisdom and compassion. I am especially grateful to the many other dharma teachers who have influenced and enriched my life, including Thich Nhat Hanh, Joseph Goldstein, Andrew Olendzki, Stephen Batchelor, and His Holiness, The Dalai Lama.

I extend my deep gratitude to the Community Meditation Center Board of Directors, volunteers, and the CMC members, who are such an important part of my life. You have placed so much in my hands, yet it is my heart that you fill to overflowing. You are my inspiration.

Thank you, Drs. Tan Bien Keem (BK) and Roger Yurt, for assisting me with medical terminology and an understanding of my condition that could be put into layman's language. Thank you, Nancy Napier, for your lucid insights into the workings of Somatic Experiencing.

Thank you, Deena Metzger and Brother David Steindl-Rast, for your gracious permission to use your work, which has added color and depth to my endeavors.

Above all, thank you, Susanna, my perfect partner, for keeping me alive so I could write and teach and enjoy all the treasures of life and our marriage.

The dharma is perfect. I, on the other hand, remain a work in progress. Any error, inaccuracy, misperception, or unskillfulness in presenting the teachings herein is strictly my doing.

A special thank you to my dear friend and agent, who believed in me and helped launch my writing career: Loretta Barrett (1940–2014).

—*Allan Lokos*
New York City, 2014

APPENDIX

A hospital is no place for a sick or injured person, but there is always the possibility that any of us might suddenly, and unexpectedly, need to be cared for in one. If so, you absolutely must have an advocate, someone who can speak up for you and see that your needs are properly and promptly addressed. One cannot overemphasize this point. If you are a patient in a hospital, you must have a supporter/champion/spokesperson.

This emphatic recommendation regarding an advocate comes from real life-and-death personal experience. Following the plane crash in which I was injured, my wife immediately assumed the role of my advocate. On six separate occasions, doctors told her that I would not survive my injuries. She refused to accept that prognosis. She fought, she demanded, she insisted, and she would not quit. When one doctor in Bangkok told her, "I'm sorry, this man is going to die," she replied, "You don't know this man." I think the truth was he did not know that woman. Recently, the *Journal of the American Geriatrics Society* published an article suggesting the creation of a new type of profession: the health fiduciary. This would be someone paid to act on behalf of those who are incapable of speaking for themselves at that time. The suggestion, in my view, is better than nothing, but my concern is that this new profession could become yet another piece in an already muddled system. Providing one's own advocate would still be the best solution.

Hospitals are incredibly complex and overly burdened

institutions. Staff are usually overworked and often fatigued, and they must function within a seriously broken health care system. For whatever reason you are hospitalized, you are not likely to be at your best, not just physically, but mentally and emotionally as well. Without someone specifically watching out for your needs, you could easily be on the wrong end of an error.

A wife/husband/partner could make a perfect advocate, but there might not be such a person in your life, in which case consider discussing the matter with an appropriate friend or colleague. A good advocate would be levelheaded, articulate, and not shy about skillfully expressing their concerns for your wellbeing. They need to be able to free up time, and in an emergency, perhaps quite a bit of time, and possibly on short notice.

One of the ways to establish this kind of relationship is to offer to make it mutual. In other words, each of you agrees to be an advocate for the other. It should be noted that even the most loving husband/wife/partner might not make the best advocate. It is wise to use skillful speech when discussing these matters. Even if your mate is not your main advocate, he or she would be the person most likely to be making important decisions for you if you become incapable of making them for yourself.

The advocate relationship as described above, while serious, is informal in nature. There are a number of legal options that would be wise to consider as well, including a "living will." This legal document is used to make known one's wishes pertaining to life-extending medical treatments. It can also be referred to as an advance directive, health care directive, or a physician's directive. A living will can be of great value since it informs your health care providers, and your family, about your wishes for life-prolonging treatment if you become unable to speak for yourself.

Patients at New York–Presbyterian Hospital are given a

paper called "Patient Information Notice—Advance Directives." It reads, in part, "[This] Hospital's policy is to honor Advance Directives that are available at the time of your visit. If you have an Advance Directive available at the time of your visit, please give it to your provider during the admission process. In the event of a medical emergency, routine medical emergency procedures will be followed unless a valid Advance Directive exists and is readily available."

During a recent hospital visit, I came across a sign at the entrance to the urology department. It is worth becoming familiar with these suggestions:

- *We encourage patients to speak up to prevent health care errors. We need your participation to help provide outstanding care.*
- *Speak up if you have questions or concerns. If you still don't understand, ask again. It's your body and you have a right to know.*
- *Pay attention to the care you get. Always make sure you get the right treatments and medicines. Don't assume anything.*
- *Educate yourself about your illness. Learn about the medical tests you will get.*
- *Ask a trusted family member or friend to be your advocate.*
- *Know what medicines you take. Know why you take them. Medicine errors are the most common health care mistakes.*
- *If you use an ambulatory care center, surgery center, office-based surgery practice, imaging center, or other type of health care organization, be sure that it has been carefully checked out.*
- *Participate in all decisions about your treatment. You are the center of your health care team.*

After the plane crash, I was taking a number of medications. My wife/advocate made a list of them, as well as the dosages, and put it in her cell phone, which she almost always has with her. A good advocate thinks of these things.

Until Christmas Day 2012, I would have thought all of this fuss about hospitals, advocates, and directives to be overreactive. I could tend to such things later. I would have been wrong. Dead wrong.

When dealing with an emotional trauma, serious injury, or illness, it is worth the time and effort to seek out and surround yourself with a team of professionals who are skillful and supportive (see page 65, The Dream Team). It is not that different from a business venture; the more competent the staff, the more we increase the likelihood of a successful outcome.

When it comes to your health, physical and mental, nothing less than the best possible outcome is acceptable. Individual needs while healing vary, but there are universal characteristics to look for when choosing the personnel who will guide and facilitate your recovery. Skill, experience, and compassion are among the most important.

Do not hesitate to request the doctor or therapist of your choice. Use terminology like, "Dr. James feels like the best fit for me," or "Lucille seems to understand my quirks better than anyone." Do not speak derogatorily about the others. Just praise the person with whom you would like to work. Unless the person you want is overbooked, you should get your first choice.

Following an injury or extended illness, it is possible that your doctor will write a script (prescription) for you so that you can work with a physical therapist. Ask the therapist questions regarding how he or she will work with you. This may not be your area of expertise, but it is your body and you have instincts. Some medical insurance covers physical therapy, so be sure to check with your provider and make sure that the therapist accepts your insurance.

Doctors and hospitals usually have a list of physical and occupational therapists they have worked with and can recommend. It is not essential that you like your therapist or, for that matter, any other member of the team, but it can make the work more enjoyable if you do, and on a particular day that can mean a lot.

One advantage to doing therapeutic work in the hospital is the amount of equipment they have at their disposal. I worked with everything from large exercise machines to tiny screws that I fastened into mini openings.

The work that the therapist does for you will be much more effective if you follow up and do the exercises at home. Ask which exercises should be done every day and which only need to be done two or three times a week. Once again, do the work. You only get one body (as far as we know) so treat it honorably, lovingly, and respectfully.

In a given moment, any member of the healing team might be "the most important." Over the long haul, however, the person who may be the most significant to our healing is he or she who guides us through the mental and emotional part of our recovery. Without a healthy, well-focused mind, true healing is unlikely.

It is not necessarily easy to find the psychotherapist, psychologist, psychiatrist, or other healing professional who is right for you. There are still circles/families in which seeking such help is seen as unacceptable, a sign of weakness, or "not what we do." The suggestion here is to look deeply within and do what is best for you. Seek a greater truth. Your mental health is supremely important. You cannot heal without it.

A therapist is in many ways like a friend, but it is a professional relationship and therapists observe certain boundaries. They will not socialize with you nor will they discuss their personal lives, unless they feel a particular anecdote could benefit you. A good therapist is nonjudgmental and is able to hear the truth beneath our hackneyed story lines. Often when the truth is mirrored back to us, it can be uncomfortable, but that is an essential part of the work if we are to heal. Likewise, they praise what is working well in our lives so as to encourage it to grow.

Many therapists are flexible with their fees and some offer sliding scales. They have entered a healing profession because they want to help.

May all beings be healthy and free from illness and pain.

SUGGESTED READING

Amaravati and Cittaviveka Buddhist Monasteries, The Nuns' Community at. *Freeing the Heart.* Great Gaddesden, UK: Amaravati Publications, 2001. Available online; a beautiful and accessible collection of diverse teachings.

Analayo. *Satipatthana: The Direct Path to Realization.* Cambridge, UK: Windhorse Publications, 2004. One of the best books available on meditation and contemplation.

Anyen Rinpoche. *Dying with Confidence: A Tibetan Buddhist's Guide to Preparing for Death.* Somerville, Mass.: Wisdom Publications, 2012. A clear, calm voice helps the reader prepare for death.

Batchelor, Stephen. *Buddhism Without Beliefs: A Contemporary Guide to Awakening.* New York: Riverhead, 1998. A short classic, highly recommended.

Bayda, Ezra. *Saying Yes to Life: (Even the Hard Parts).* Somerville, Mass.: Wisdom Publications, 2005. Easy-to-grasp inspiration for each day.

Bhikkhu Bodhi. *In the Buddha's Words: An Anthology of Discourses from the Pali Canon.* Somerville, Mass.: Wisdom Publications, 2005. A wonderful introduction to the Buddha's teaching in his own words.

Boccio, Frank Jude. *Mindfulness Yoga: The Awakened Union of Breath, Body, and Mind.* Somerville, Mass.: Wisdom Publications, 1993. Integrates Buddhist teachings with asana yoga practice.

Boorstein, Sylvia. *Happiness Is an Inside Job: Practicing for a Joyful Life.* New York: Ballantine Books, 2008 (reprint). Teachings on how to move away from anger, anxiety, and confusion into calmness, clarity, and joy.

Brach, Tara. *Radical Acceptance: Embracing Your Life with the Heart of a Buddha.* New York: Bantam, 2004. Poetry and kind advice from an experienced psychotherapist and Buddhist meditation teacher; deserving of its popularity.

_____. *True Refuge: Finding Peace and Freedom in Your Own Awakened Heart.* New York: Bantam, 2013. Drawing on recent findings in neuroscience to offer heartfelt insight; lovely and wise.

Chah, Ajahn. *Being Dharma: The Essence of the Buddha's Teachings.* Boston: Shambhala, 2001. With a foreword by Jack Kornfield; contains many of Ajahn Chah's memorable teachings in condensed form.

_____. *A Still Forest Pool: The Insight Meditation of Achaan Chah.* Edited by Jack Kornfield and Paul Breiter. Wheaton, Ill.: Quest Books, 2004. A master teacher shares his quiet, joyful message.

Chödrön, Pema. *Comfortable with Uncertainty: 108 Teachings on Cultivating Fearlessness and Compassion.* Boston: Shambhala, 2003. Short readings to help cultivate compassion and awareness from a popular teacher/author.

_____. *The Places That Scare You: A Guide to Fearlessness in Difficult Times.* Boston: Shambhala, 2002. Tools to deal with the problems and difficulties that life throws our way.

Chödrön, Thubten. *Working with Anger.* Boston: Snow Lion Publications, 2001. Insights into anger, with helpful suggestions.

Dalai Lama. *The Dalai Lama's Little Book of Inner Peace: The Essential Life and Teachings.* Newburyport, Mass.: Hampton Roads Publishing, 2009. Advice on how to live a peaceful and fulfilling life.

Epstein, Mark. *Thoughts Without a Thinker: Psychotherapy from a Buddhist Perspective.* New York: Basic Books, 1995. An integration of Western psychology and Buddhist wisdom.

Glassman, Bernie. *Bearing Witness: A Zen Master's Lessons in Making Peace.* New York: Harmony/Bell Tower, 1999. Teaching stories illustrate ways of making peace.

Goldstein, Joseph. *Mindfulness: A Practical Guide to Awakening.* Louisville, Colo.: Sounds True, 2013. From Goldstein's forty years of teaching and practice comes this monumental work focused on spiritual awakening.

Goleman, Daniel. *The Meditative Mind: The Varieties of Meditative Experience.*

New York: Tarcher, 1996 (reprint). A first-rate introduction to meditation.

Gunaratana, Bhante Henepola. *Mindfulness in Plain English.* Somerville, Mass.: Wisdom Publications, 1996. Regarded by many as one of the very best introductions to Buddhist meditation, it is a gem.

Hanson, Rick. *Buddha's Brain: The Practical Neuroscience of Happiness, Love, and Wisdom.* Oakland, Calif.: New Harbinger Publications, 2009. Uses neuroscience and mindfulness practice to tap the potential of your brain; excellent for all levels.

Herrigel, Eugen. *Zen in the Art of Archery.* New York: Vintage Books, 1999 (1948). A perennial classic and most worthy.

Hillesum, Etty. *Etty Hillesum: An Interrupted Life: The Diaries, 1941–1943; and Letters from Westerbork.* New York: Picador, 1996. Testifies to the possibility of awareness and compassion even in the most devastating challenge to one's humanity.

Hoblitzelle, Olivia Ames. *Ten Thousand Joys & Ten Thousand Sorrows: A Couple's Journey Through Alzheimer's.* New York: Tarcher, 2010 (reprint). A beautiful and heartbreaking account of a couple's experience with a devastating illness.

Housden, Roger. *Ten Poems to Change Your Life.* New York: Harmony, 2001. Shows how poetry illuminates eternal feelings and desires.

Kabat-Zinn, Jon. *Full Catastrophe Living: Using the Wisdom of Your Body and Mind to Face Stress, Pain, and Illness.* McHenry, Ill.: Delta, 1990 (reprint). Shows how to use natural methods to heal your body, mind, and spirit.

————. *Wherever You Go, There You Are: Mindfulness Meditation in Everyday Life.* New York: Hyperion, 2005 (1994). Groundbreaking bestseller that can change a life.

Ko-I Bastis, Madeline. *Peaceful Dwelling: Meditations for Healing and Living.* Boston: Tuttle Publishing, 2000. Meditations for healing a variety of medical, psychological, or spiritual ailments.

Kornfield, Jack. *A Path with Heart: A Guide Through the Perils and Promises of*

Spiritual Life. New York: Bantam, 1993. Advice garnered from twenty-five years of teaching the path of awakening.

Levine, Peter. *Waking the Tiger: Healing Trauma.* Berkeley, Calif.: North Atlantic Books, 1997. Normalizes the symptoms of trauma and the steps needed to heal them.

Levine, Stephen. *A Year to Live: How to Live This Year as If It Were Your Last.* New York: Bell Tower, 1998. Teaches how to live each moment as if it were our last.

Lokos, Allan. *Patience: The Art of Peaceful Living.* New York: Tarcher/Penguin, 2012. An in-depth and accessible exploration of this vitally important virtue.

Lozoff, Bo. *It's a Meaningful Life: It Just Takes Practice.* New York: Penguin Compass, 2001 (reprint). Posits that compassion is at the root of happiness.

McLeod, Ken. *Wake Up to Your Life: Discovering the Buddhist Path of Attention.* New York: HarperOne, 2002. A thorough guide for someone exploring Buddhist views on their own.

Maitreya, Ananda (translator). *The Dhammapada.* Berkeley, Calif.: Parallax Press, 1995. A concise guide to a better life; profound. There are other excellent translations.

Markova, Dawna. *I Will Not Die an Unlived Life: Reclaiming Purpose and Passion.* Newburyport, Mass.: Conari Press, 2000. How to be more intimate with the value and purpose of life.

Muller, Wayne. *How Then Shall We Live?: Four Simple Questions That Reveal the Beauty and Meaning of Our Lives.* New York: Bantam, 1997. Contemplations, practices, poems, and teachings from the great wisdom traditions.

————. *Legacy of the Heart: The Spiritual Advantages of a Painful Childhood.* New York: Touchstone, 1993. Uncovering spiritual strength in the scars of childhood.

Napier, Nancy. *Sacred Practices for Conscious Living.* New York: W. W. Norton, 1997. A worldview focused on the blending of spiritual and material realities.

Nepo, Mark. *The Book of Awakening: Having the Life You Want by Being Present to the Life You Have.* Newburyport, Mass.: Conari Press, 2000. The best daybook, and an Oprah favorite.

Nhat Hanh, Thich. *Being Peace.* Berkeley, Calif.: Parallax Press, 2005 (2nd ed.). Beautiful, gentle words from a beautiful, gentle teacher.

————. *Thich What Hanh: Essential Writings.* Maryknoll, N.Y.: Orbis Books, 2001. Snippets of the Vietnamese master's work; essential reading.

————. *The Heart of the Buddha's Teaching: Transforming Suffering into Peace, Joy and Liberation.* New York: Broadway Books, 1999. The core teachings of Buddhism offered with heart.

Olendzki, Andrew. *Unlimiting Mind: The Radically Experiential Psychology of Buddhism.* Somerville, Mass.: Wisdom Publications, 2010. Sophisticated, scholarly, and accessible insights into Buddhist psychology.

Palmer, Parker. *Let Your Life Speak: Listening for the Voice of Vocation.* San Francisco: Jossey-Bass, 1999. Invites us to listen to the inner teacher and follow it toward a sense of meaning and purpose.

Pandita, Sayadaw U. *In This Very Life: The Liberation Teachings of the Buddha.* Somerville, Mass.: Wisdom Publications, 1995. The path to liberation as laid out by a Burmese master.

Ram Dass. *Still Here: Embracing Aging, Changing, and Dying.* New York: Riverhead Books, 2001. Addresses the big questions of peace and purpose.

————. and Paul Gorman. *How Can I Help?: Stories and Reflections on Service.* New York: Alfred A. Knopf, 1985. A guide for friends and families trying to meet each other's needs.

Remen, Rachel Naomi. *My Grandfather's Blessings: Stories of Strength, Refuge, and Belonging.* New York: Riverhead, 2001. Stories to remind us of the power of kindness and the joys of life.

Rosenberg, Larry. *Breath by Breath: The Liberating Practice of Insight Meditation.* Boston: Shambhala, 2004. Makes insight meditation practice accessible for westerners.

Salzberg, Sharon. *Faith: Trusting Your Own Deepest Experience.* New York: Riverhead, 2003. A guide to understanding the healing qualities of faith by one of the world's most loved teachers.

_____. *Real Happiness: The Power of Meditation: A 28-Day Program.* New York: Workman, 2012. A *New York Times* bestseller that is thorough and easy to follow; first rate.

Sogyal Rinpoche. *The Tibetan Book of Living and Dying.* San Francisco: HarperSanFrancisco, 2012 (rev. ed.). Monumental, indispensable, and challenging introduction to Tibetan Buddhism.

Surya Das, Lama. *Awakening the Buddha Within: Tibetan Wisdom for the Western World.* New York: Broadway Books, 1998 (reprint). Awaken to who we really are to lead a more compassionate and balanced life.

Suzuki, Shunryu. *Zen Mind, Beginner's Mind.* Boston: Shambhala, 2011 (1970). A modern Zen classic; the basics and so much more.

Retreat Centers and Meditation Centers

Retreat centers generally offer residential retreats of a few days to several months. Meditation centers may offer training in meditation, practice, teachings, and daylong retreats. For an extensive listing of retreat centers in the United States, see retreatfinder.com.

Against the Stream Buddhist Meditation Society
4300 Melrose Avenue
Los Angeles, CA 90029
againstthestream.org
323-665-4300
Noah Levine
Vipassana teaching and practice

Barre Center for Buddhist Studies
149 Lockwood Road
Barre, MA 01005
bcbsdharma.org
978-355-2347
bcbs@dharma.org
The study center offers a variety of courses, workshops, retreats, and
    self-study programs to further research, study, and practice. BCBS
    provides a bridge between study and practice, between scholarly
    understanding and meditative insight.

Blue Cliff Monastery

3 Mindfulness Road
Pine Bush, NY 12566
bluecliffmonastery.org

845-733-4959
office@bluecliffmonastery.org

Blue Cliff Monastery in upstate New York (two hours from New York
City) is an extension of Plum Village meditation center in France,
founded by the Zen monk Thich Nhat Hanh.

Cambridge Insight Meditation Center

331 Broadway
Cambridge, MA 02139
cambridgeinsight.org

617-441-9038

Guiding teachers are Larry Rosenberg, Narayan Helen Liebenson, and
Michael Grady.

Insight Meditation integrated with contemplative and daily life
practice.

Community Meditation Center

5 West 86th Street
New York, NY 10024
cmcnewyork.org

212-787-7272

Allan Lokos, guiding teacher, plus guest teachers

Weekly sessions grounded in the Buddhist Theravada tradition offered
on Sunday mornings and Wednesday evenings include meditation,
dharma talk, and discussion. One-day retreats. Appropriate for
beginners and advanced meditators.

Garrison Institute

14 Mary's Way, Route 9D

Garrison, NY 10524

garrisoninstitute.org

845-424-4800

A beautifully renovated Capuchin monastery on the Hudson River fifty minutes north of New York City, the Garrison Institute is a nonsectarian organization dedicated to the intersection of contemplation and engaged action. They offer a variety of retreats of varying lengths.

Great Vow Zen Monastery—Part of the Zen Community of Oregon

P.O. Box 188

Clatskanie, OR 97016

zendust.org/monastery

503-728-0654

Teachers Jan Chozen Bays, Roshi

A residential monastery with public programs. Soto and Rinzai Zen with Theravada ethics and Dzogchen view.

Insight Meditation Society and The Forest Refuge

1230 Pleasant Street

Barre, MA 01005

dharma.org

978-355-4378

rc@dharma.org

Founded by Joseph Goldstein, Jack Kornfield, and Sharon Salzberg, IMS is a spiritual refuge for all who seek freedom of mind and heart. They offer meditation retreats rooted in the Theravada Buddhist teachings of ethics, concentration, and wisdom.

The Forest Refuge is for experienced meditators wanting a longer individual retreat.

Kripalu
57 Interlaken Road
Stockbridge, MA 01262
kripalu.org
800-741-7353
Located in the Berkshire Mountains of western Massachusetts, Kripalu
is the largest retreat center for yoga, health, and holistic living in
North America.

The Mountain Hermitage
P.O. Box 807
Ranchos de Taos, NM 87557
mountainhermitage.org
575-758-0633
Marcia Rose, guiding teacher; and visiting teachers
Vipassana, concentration, Brahma Viharas study and practice, and
creativity

New York Insight Meditation Center
28 West 27th Street
New York, NY 10001
nyimc.org
212-213-4802
Gina Sharp, guiding teacher; staff teachers; and guest teachers

Omega Institute Daily programs throughout the year
150 Lake Drive
Rhinebeck, NY 12572
eomega.org
877-944-2002; 845-266-4444
The Omega Institute for Holistic Studies offers programs on its

campus in Rhinebeck, New York, and at other locations around the world. The focus is on health and wellness, spiritual growth, and self-awareness.

San Francisco Zen Center

300 Page Street
San Francisco, CA 94102
sfzc.org
415-863-3136
One of the largest Buddhist communities outside Asia, offers daily meditation, regular monastic retreats and practice periods, classes, lectures, and workshops. All are welcome.

Seattle Insight Meditation Society

2729 6th Avenue South
Seattle, Washington 98134
seattleinsight.org
206-366-2111
Rodney Smith, guiding teacher
Introductory and ongoing Insight Meditation classes, weekend nonresidential retreats, and online dharma talks

Shambhala Mountain Center

151 Shambhala Way
Red Feather Lakes, CO 80545
shambhalamountain.org
888-788-7221
callcenter@shambhalamountain.org
This northern Colorado center offers meditation, yoga, and other practices.

Southern Dharma Retreat Center
1661 West Road
Hot Springs, NC 28743
southerndharma.org
828-622-7112
southerndharma@earthlink.net
This interfaith retreat center in the Blue Ridge Mountains of western
    North Carolina hosts retreats in a variety of spiritual traditions.

Spirit Rock Meditation Center
5000 Sir Francis Drake Boulevard
Woodacre, CA 94973
spiritrock.org
415-488-0164
Spirit Rock is dedicated to the teachings of the Buddha in the
    Vipassana tradition. The practice of Insight Meditation is at the
    heart of all activities. They offer silent meditation retreats, as well
    as classes, trainings, and dharma study.

Upaya Zen Center
1404 Cerro Gordo Road
Santa Fe, NM 87501
upaya.org
505-986-8518
Roshi Joan Halifax, PhD
Meditation, dharma talks, retreats, training

Zen Mountain Monastery
P.O. Box 197
Mount Tremper, NY 12457
zmm.mro.org
845-688-2228
In New York's Catskill Mountains, retreats and residential programs
    are offered.

If you enjoyed this book, visit

www.tarcherbooks.com

and sign up for Tarcher's e-newsletter to receive
special offers, giveaway promotions, and
information on hot upcoming releases.

TARCHER
PENGUIN

Great Lives Begin with Great Ideas

Connect with the Tarcher Community

. . .

Stay in touch with favorite authors!
Enter weekly contests!
Read exclusive excerpts!
Voice your opinions!

Follow us

 Tarcher Books

@TarcherBooks

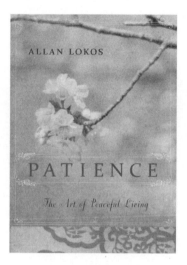

"This book, both practical and profound, is a wonderful demonstration of just how to bring patience and a new way of being right into our daily lives. It is filled with insight, warmth, and compassion."

—Sharon Salzberg, author of *Real Happiness* and *Lovingkindness*

978-1-58542-900-4 $14.95

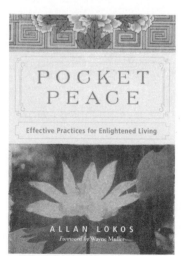

"Stress is a sure happiness killer, but the antidote just might be *Pocket Peace* by Allan Lokos . . . Lokos brings a calming Buddhist slant to urban angst, doling out creative, easy-as-pie practices (choose a belonging you really like and give it away to discover how you feel about attachment issues) to help soothe your way, offering another great option for turning over new pages in your life."

—*The Boston Globe*

978-1-58542-781-9 $13.95